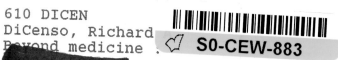

BEYOND MEDICINE

EXPLORING A NEW WAY OF THINKING

Dr. Richard A. DiCenso

Matrix Transformation
Virginia Beach, VA

Published by Matrix Transformation
372 South Independence Blvd., Suite 105
Virginia Beach, VA 23452

Publisher's Cataloging-in-Publication Data
DiCenso, Richard A.

Beyond medicine : exploring a new way of thinking / Richard A. DiCenso – Virginia Beach, VA : Matrix Transformation, 2006.

p. ; cm.
ISBN: 0-9670761-1-0
ISBN13: 978-0-9670761-1-9

1. Alternative medicine. 2. Health. 3. Self-care, Health. I. Title.

R733 .D53 2005
610—dc22   2005938192

Book production and coordination by Jenkins Group, Inc. • www.BookPublishing.com
Cover design by Karen Moscoffian
Interior design by Debbie Sidman

Printed in the United States of America
10 09 08 07 06 • 5 4 3 2 1

Dedication

"The average, healthy, well-adjusted adult gets up at seven-thirty in the morning feeling just plain terrible."

—Jean Kerr, author

Dedication is not what others expect of you, it is what you can give to others. And so, I offer this book to you, dedicated to the thousands of pilgrims roaming the paths of self-directed wellness. So, too, I dedicate this book to the unwell that have yet to recognize that they cannot escape the responsibility of tomorrow by evading it today. And finally, I dedicate this book to my greatest teacher, the one and the many without whom none of this would be possible.

My agenda for presenting the material contained within the pages of this book is to provoke thoughtful insight and stimulate awareness. In so doing, it is my hope that each person who reads this book will seek to aspire to his or her own personal best. To alter your experience consciously and deliberately, you must know three things. Firstly, you must recognize where you are. Secondly, you must know where you want to be. And thirdly, you must know how to get from here to there. The purpose of this book is to provide you with the tools for accomplishing all three of these goals.

In dedicating this book to you, I pass along the task of exploring the information herein with nothing more than your attention and an open mind. Having done that, I challenge you to choose what is appropriate for your life and apply it. Similarly, I propose that you discard that which does not resonate true for you. In either case, I remind you that he who hesitates is not only lost, but is miles from the next exit.

I offer you the tools for transformation, extracted from my own personal and professional life experience. This is a reference manual for looking at things differently.

Acknowledgments

Creative projects require an enormous collaboration with trusted allies and supporters. Needless to say, there are typically dozens of individuals involved in preparing an undertaking of this nature for public consumption. Of course, there are the publishers, editors, book designers, proofreaders, graphic designers, and project managers. But I would be remiss if I did not single out a few very special individuals without whom *Beyond Medicine* would not exist.

First and foremost, there is my partner, best friend and biggest fan, Karen Moscoffian. She has been ever-present throughout the planning, development, and execution of every phase leading up to the completion of this book. Her touch is in every detail down to the type style, layout, design and colors. But most of all her expertise is memorialized in the design and presentation of the cover. Kudos Karen and thank you!

David Holt, M.D., has been a friend and ally throughout the re-writes, editing, and proofreading process. At each step he was present to offer support, advice, encouragement, and valuable insights. Thank you David. Eleanor Woloy, M.D., was gracious enough to review the entire early manuscript and submit the kind words on the back cover.

And to you, my patients, supporters, investors, and friends, thank you for everything. Special thanks to Jill, Myron, Kevin, Shirley, Rose, Alan, Lynn, Emily, Tom, Marge, Bill and Bob.

Contents

Foreword

There is a revolution going on in American healthcare today. I am not talking about the technological advances that are bringing us more amazing treatments for illnesses, or the extraordinary new medical imaging devices that allow doctors to view inside virtually any area of our bodies. Neither am I referring to the explosive progress in the field of genetics that has cracked the human genome and soon promises cures for diseases for which no effective treatments exist.

I am talking about the revolution in *alternative health*. This term encompasses much more than alternative practices such as acupuncture and naturopathic medicine. It goes well beyond vitamins and herbs, visualization techniques, and aromatherapy. It fundamentally involves a profound change in the way Americans perceive their own health and the established medical healthcare system.

Americans no longer trust their healthcare system. They have come to question what their doctors and the medical establishment have been telling them all these years: things they have always accepted on faith without questioning. Increasingly, they see their physicians as being too busy to take a personal interest in their health. They recognize a medical establishment that has shown itself to be all too eager to sell them on the latest prescription drug or invasive diagnostic procedure, only to take their money and run. All too often, they find themselves left with no substantive improvement in their health. Worse yet, they are plagued with the harmful side effects of medication or surgical complications, which lead to the necessity of greater reliance on a healthcare system that failed them in the first place. Ultimately, they find themselves left with a bewildering array of healthcare choices and no one they can trust to turn to for help in navigating this maze.

People are taking more responsibility for their health. They are becoming informed consumers when it comes to their healthcare choices. They are looking beyond conventional medicine for answers to their healthcare needs. This area, beyond medicine, is sometimes referred to as *alternative health*, or *complimentary medicine*. But it is much more than just that. It is the world of all things implied in these terms, to be sure. But more fundamentally, it is a world of choices, which give us far greater freedoms and almost frighteningly complex options to control our own health potential, and ultimately our own lives. Traversing this world leads to a new way of perceiving ourselves, our bodies, and our relationship with the world around us. The old models of living the American dream, getting regular check-ups with the family doctor, and growing old gracefully no longer seem to be relevant. People are seeking to redefine their relationship with this world of health choices, but they are finding it difficult to know where to begin, what it is that they really want, or what they truly need.

This book explores this world beyond medicine. The author, Dr. Richard DiCenso, begins by exploring the nature of reality and the *realms* that define our relationship with the world around and within us. You might wonder what a philosophical discussion like this has to do with illness and health. The answer is *everything*.

As Dr. DiCenso so carefully explains, reality *is* actually fluid and changeable. Within the virtual realm of our consciousness, reality *is* pretty much what you choose to make it. Not just your interpretation of reality, but *reality* itself. This means that with respect to the body-mind connection, what you think becomes what you feel and what you believe becomes who you are. We have all heard things like this coming from sources such as Dr. Norman Vincent Peale in *The Power of Positive Thinking,* as well as from the numerous self-help gurus and get-rich-quick hucksters. The end product is that we come away thinking that people can convince themselves of pretty much anything, if they want to. There is a thread of truth running through all of these diverse sources. The net effect has been to condition us to believe that it is all just pretending, and that reality is really still just, well ... reality. Thus, we each stay within the static and unyielding versions of who we are and what we can and cannot feel. Comforted in this familiarity, we are isolated from change.

In this book, Dr. DiCenso opens the doorways to change. To do so, he gives us a guided tour of the virtual realm where reality is infinitely changeable. In many ways, Dr. DiCenso is the Carl Sagan of the human mind-body science-philosophy. In reading this work, I am at times reminded of sitting in a vast planetarium with the astronomer-guide leading me on a journey through the heavens as they unfold in splendor before my eyes.

I must confess that at times I had difficulty understanding some of what I was reading. I found myself rereading sentences, or even whole paragraphs, over and over until I was satisfied I understood what Dr. DiCenso was explaining. In fact, the harder I struggled to pin down what I was reading, the more elusive this understanding became. Finally I realized, I wasn't just reading the material, I was trying to change it to conform to my own perception of reality. Once I understood this, I relaxed and actually began enjoying what I was reading. To my amazement, I also understood it much better. I am reminded of the Beatles' lyric: *"Turn off your mind, relax and float down stream."* So I urge the reader to enjoy the ride as Dr. DiCenso leads us on an amazing journey through the mind-body continuum and the collective mind we all seem to sense, but often have no words to describe. Dr. DiCenso gives us the words, the pictures and the road map to follow, while navigating this journey on our own.

Two key elements of this roadmap to personal change are Dr. DiCenso's *caveats* and his concept of *Vicious Cycle Disorders*. The caveats are the pearls of wisdom gleaned from his thirty years of experience in the clinical application of diverse disciplines. They are simple, but profound, truths that are held to be self-evident and which serve as signposts to guide us along our way.

Dr. DiCenso's concept of Vicious Cycle Disorders beautifully describes the self-perpetuating nature of many of the unrelenting burdens we carry in life. These burdens include the chronic diseases that are so often lifestyle-dependent, as well as the undiagnosed illnesses represented by vague symptoms. Like a scratch on the record album of our personal realities, the Vicious Cycle Disorder keeps skipping. It causes the recurrence of the same

thoughts, behaviors, and physiologic responses that lead to the same negative outcomes over and over again. Vicious Cycle Disorders undercut the
homeostatic processes that maintain balance in our lives, and sabotage the
self-healing capabilities of our bodies. Dr. DiCenso shows us how to identify these processes and explains how we can effectively deal with them.

This is an important book for many reasons. It should be on the required
reading list for all alternative and conventional healthcare providers who
seek to help their patients unravel the mysteries of their symptoms and
change their lives. By establishing the biophysical basis of the body-mind
connection, Dr. DiCenso closes the gap that separates medical and naturopathic sciences. He creates a theoretical framework in which treatment
approaches from both fields can be brought to bear on a particular health
problem. This book is also important for those individuals who wish to better understand themselves and others around them. Dr. DiCenso has the
unique gift of seeing clearly through the haze that separates each of us in
our individual perceptions of reality. Not only is he able to see plainly into
this realm of virtual reality, but he is also able to guide us through it and
show us how to navigate this world on our own. I have read no other book
of philosophy, Eastern mysticism or Western psychotherapeutics that
comes close to such clarity of vision in explaining how consciousness
works in directing the mind-body relationship.

David B. Holt, M.D.

Preface

Do you *experience* radiant health? Do you have peace of mind? Is your personal life fulfilling? Is your professional life rewarding? Do you look forward to each new day? Do you experience abundance and prosperity in your day-to-day interactions? Do you feel secure, cared for and loved? Are you living your dream? Are you happy?

If you answered no to any or all of these questions, you may be suffering from a Vicious Cycle Disorder (VCD). At any given time, approximately 20 percent of the population endures unresolved symptoms of a life out of balance. These symptoms frequently present themselves as an overall lack of well-being. They are confirmed by everything from constant headaches and low energy to financial stress and tumultuous relationships.

The symptoms are usually chronic and low-grade, earmarked by a lack of objective findings and negative test results. They are frequently accompanied by recurrent feelings. These feelings rarely appear to be related to how we feel physically. They present themselves in the form of remorse, depression, anger, resentment, lack of self-esteem, loneliness, worry, abandonment, insecurity, frustration, and anxiety. Often, they are experienced as chronic pain of unknown, or at least insubstantial, origins.

If you are experiencing constant symptoms that concern you and interfere with your enjoyment of life, you may be suffering from VCD. Having served as clinical director and program administrator in numerous healthcare facilities over the last twenty-five years I have seen countless patients suffering needlessly from these same kinds of symptoms. If you've been told that all your tests are negative, your symptoms are normal for your age, they will go away in time, you'll have to learn to live with them, we can't find anything wrong, or they're all in your head, VCD may be at the root of all your problems.

The good news is that there is hope. You can discover and expose the cause of VCD. Once identified, it can be modified or eliminated. The bad news is that you have created it all yourself. Any behavior repeated to excess can be the cause of VCD. This can include, but is not limited to, the activities we perform, the habits we have acquired, the foods that we eat, or any other area of physical engagement. Any repetitive thought, word, or action can cause VCD. In *Beyond Medicine,* I will show you how VCD develops and what you can do about it.

Sometimes we get lost in the activities of daily life that demand our attention. Sometimes we fail to remember who we really are and what our lives really represent. Sometimes we forget the hopes, dreams, and aspirations of days gone by. Sometimes we lose sight of our dreams. Sometimes we forget to dream. Sometimes we simply don't know how to dream.

Researchers estimate that humans have approximately 60,000 thoughts per day. They suggest that these thoughts determine each person's reality experience. The problem appears to be in the nature and quality of thoughts repeatedly entertained on a daily basis. The challenge is to identify these thoughts, acknowledge them as self-created and change them. Changing the experience of life can be as simple as changing one's mind about the thoughts regularly hosted. It can literally be as simple as changing how and what you think.

However, to change your mind you must become aware of the process that is used to create the thoughts you think. Assume that paying attention to something energizes your intention to experience it. In other words, your intention to have a particular experience produces a transformation from where you are to where you want to be. Then, to truly transform, you must first become attentive to the source from which experiences originate. This process requires an assessment of your thoughts. Thoughts are things that materialize from the unseen realm and provide the basis for everything you experience. In the final analysis, you have chosen to experience the thoughts that you think.

Becoming "whole" again involves the process of consciously employing free will, or self-actualizing, at the level of thought. Unfortunately, this skill is rarely encouraged and frequently suppressed in early childhood as individual personalities emerge. The unlimited potential of youth is refined out of existence, as society imposes instruction on how to limit the experience of reality. *What* to think is taught in lieu of *how* to think.

Yet, the urges persist, as censored longings transmit a desire to experience pleasure and avoid pain. Memories of the past fuel a desire for the future, and patterns of behavior designed to satisfy the need for fulfillment are cultivated. Subsequent actions produce experiences that create the desire to either repeat or avoid the results of these actions. That which "feels good" becomes an enticement to experience those things again. That which is unpleasant creates a desire to abstain from experiencing those feelings or activities.

However, engaging in activities that "feel good," but are fundamentally harmful and counterproductive, distracts from the ultimate goal of fulfillment. Learning how to identify these behaviors and modify them at the level of conception can engender a dynamic, rewarding, and satisfying way of life. Not doing so will lead to more of what you are already experiencing.

Beyond Medicine is a guide to the future of the moment in which all things exist and are available for the asking. Learning how to ask is the only skill required to return to a condition of abundant blessings. The life you have always imagined is as close as your next thought.

Introduction

A well-known saying professes that the journey of 1,000 miles begins with a single step. *Beyond Medicine* is that first step, providing a road map to the realization of dreams. In the pages that follow, the journey from here to there will be revealed. In my previous book, *A Question of Balance*, I established a framework for exploring human existence. The purpose of that work was to assist in an expanded understanding of the concept that life is multifaceted in nature. In *Beyond Medicine*, we will travel further to explore the multidimensional distinctiveness of existence.

■ Realm Consciousness

Human beings function in three primary realms: the physical, biochemical, and psycho-emotional-spiritual. Because this final realm is wholly unseen and essentially intangible, I refer to it as the "virtual." Each realm has numerous sub-categories of distinction. These sub-categories exist primarily as speculative aids to assist in understanding the purpose of the whole person they embody.

Unless balance exists among and within the realms, day-to-day life reflects discrepancies in the form of physical ailments, physiological dysfunction, and/or, emotional distress. More commonly, imbalance among the three realms expresses itself as a life wrought with fear, doubt, anxiety, depression, and many other possible symptoms of an imbalance in the unseen, virtual realm.

Technically, the unseen realm includes the biochemical realm as well. But the biochemical realm is far from unseen. There are a myriad of tools with which to examine and observe the behavior of this realm. The biochemical aspect of human experience is actually a transitional reflection of the interaction between the physical and virtual realms. It can frequently provide powerful clues as to where the cause of a discomfort is rooted. It may support the suspicion of a technical malfunction or a functional imbalance. It may also simply be the result of an emotional turmoil originating in the virtual realm that expresses itself through biochemistry. Understanding how to interpret what is seen is a critical aid to implementing an appropriate antidote.

The physical realm is more clearly appreciated as an individual entity. It appears to stand alone. Reliably, it is a testament to our genetics, environment, and our lifestyle choices. This realm is intimately woven into the fabric of the other two realms, despite its apparent self-governing individuality.

Given that the physical body is a means of transportation between birth and death, it functions exclusively in the material realm. Consequently, it is also subject to the linear laws of cause and effect. Nonetheless, it remains the ultimate outward manifestation of thoughts and activities. When gratification is experienced from eating too much food, or too much of the wrong types of foods, well-documented consequences occur. Too little or too much sleep, exercise, or water, can generate excessive stresses. The outcome can be tragic and somewhat predictable.

Likewise, if the essential nature of the virtual realm is ignored, a life of routines and random experiences ensues. Dwelling in the imaginative promise of the virtual, while repeatedly sowing seeds of anger, negativity, fear, or doubt, generates fruit that manifests itself in a physical experience beyond the temporary pleasure of a familiar behavior. Oftentimes, these repeated activities are rooted in some form of lack, or insufficiency. They can be associated with a lack of self-esteem, a lack of security, a lack of confidence, or any other form of acquired or imagined deficiency. Typically, the lack eventually leads to self-defeating behavior that produces an expectation of failure and disappointment that ultimately results in a self-fulfilling prophecy of unworthiness.

■ CHAPTER ONE ■

Emergence of the Caveats

"You cannot travel within and stand still without."

—JAMES LANE ALLEN

The working dynamic that initially emerged from my heightened exposure to realm consciousness gave rise to the notion that human existence involves far more than just a body. To thoroughly address the needs
of the whole person, it became obvious that I must at least explore, if not
understand, all three realms. This prototype evolved over a period of years
of frustrating encounters with patients I saw in my practice. These patients
were experiencing symptoms that refused to yield to what seemed like an
obvious course of therapeutic intervention.

Having been fortunate enough to perform a portion of my internship in
a prestigious hospital environment in Beverly Hills, CA, I meandered
through a vast succession of credentialing programs in search of solutions
to these ongoing healthcare issues. Following my graduation from chiropractic and acupuncture schools I scoured the disciplines of everything

from homeopathy, applied kinesiology, iridology, movement therapy, meditation, yoga, and jin shin do to clinical nutrition, human biochemistry, and forensics. After I graduated from the Spine Research Institute in San Diego and was credentialed as an expert in soft tissue trauma, I felt secure in my understanding of the evolution of physical trauma and associated symptoms. However, following my training as a chiropractic forensic examiner, I felt I finally possessed a tool that could help me to understand the dynamics of more exotic healthcare concerns that had less than obvious causes associated with them.

Over the last thirty years, I have had the opportunity to develop and administer programs at some of the most esteemed healthcare facilities in the country. In my role as clinical director of Advanced Therapeutics Virginia in Virginia Beach, VA, I was driven to discover several characteristics and circumstances to explain and assist in resolving inequities that involved the whole person. This newfound awareness produced a number of precepts and guidelines that I came to embrace as caveats. These caveats were born of the questions I encountered in my day-to-day interactions with people at my clinic who felt that something was just not right.

Plagued by unanswered questions, I felt overwhelmed. I was fully aware that there could be no question without an answer, and no problem without a solution. Nevertheless, how could I possibly know these answers? How could I solve these problems? How could I possibly help these people? Simple questions from my patients continued to plague me, such as, "Why do I hurt all over?" "Why am I not sleeping at night?" "Why won't my headaches go away?" More complex issues surfaced, such as, "Why do I continue to be depressed?" "Why do I have no energy?" "Why won't my skin clear up?" "Why do I just not feel well?"

Of course, it did not end there. Countless other patients who were suffering from commonplace dysfunctions were simply not responding to anything. There was high blood pressure, low blood pressure, diabetes, thyroid problems, irritable bowel syndrome, diarrhea, constipation, and arthritis, not to mention, infertility, chronic infections, fibromyalgia, chronic fatigue, attention deficit disorder, and acid reflux. Not surprisingly, I had not even begun to explore the world of chronic degenerative and autoimmune diseases, let alone the cultural stigmas of obesity, heart conditions, and cancer.

As I delved deeper into these problems, a series of caveats began to emerge. These caveats helped me to see beyond physical symptoms, and allowed me to realize that the human experience involved a multifaceted dynamic that included the physical, biochemical, and psycho-emotional-spiritual realms. The seven caveats I discovered include:

- Anything can cause anything.
- For every action, there is a reaction.
- Everything works.
- There are no panaceas.
- When all you have is a hammer, everything looks like a nail.
- When you hear hoof beats, look for horses.
- Everything is what it isn't.

■ The First Caveat: Anything Can Cause Anything

The first and most powerful caveat to emerge dictated awareness and perspective more so than a resolve of specific issues. That caveat is simply, "Anything can cause anything." A subsequent insight posed another question. If anything can cause anything, then how is it possible to know what is causing what? At this time, my studies were limited to trying to solve a physical problem with a physical solution. By this time, I had acknowledged a possible interaction with the other spheres of influence. But I had no real clue as to how I might evaluate them or what to do if I suspected involvement of one or the other possibilities.

For that reason, I initiated a study of the laws of cause and effect and discovered a seemingly illogical and disturbing predicament. Cause and effect are predictable in the physical realm, which includes everything that can be experienced with the five senses. This is the realm of firm boundaries containing matter, objects, and three-dimensional existence. This is the domain of the material world. This realm is made up of day-to-day experiences.

In fact, the laws of cause and effect govern the physical world. It is possible to determine how far we can travel on a tank of gas, what time the sun will rise and set, how long it will take a meal to cook, how many calories must be expended to burn a pound of fat, how much pressure is required to separate a paper towel, or how much our monthly payment must be increased to reduce a mortgage and get out of debt. Regardless, finding the anything that could cause the something I was confronted with became a fundamental premise for the working model that would allow me to directly resolve these illusive symptom complexes.

■ The Second Caveat: For Every Action There Is a Reaction

As I attempted to apply these same methods of analysis to the unseen realms, I encountered a small problem. They do not work the same way and are far less predictable. Even less predictable was my attempt to correlate cause and effect between or among realms. Regardless of this detail, these methods did work to the extent that they unveiled another tier of knowledge in the form of another caveat: "For every action there is a reaction." But there was a fly in the ointment. It was not just only or always an equal and opposite reaction. How could this be possible? On closer inspection, the individual realms displayed unique characteristics that further defined an orderliness of function. Yet a frustrating randomness pervaded their function. These realms flourished as individual entities, but somehow interacted to bring about life's experiences.

For example, the biochemical realm is transitional in nature. Certain aspects of this realm are tangible and observable, while others just seem to unexpectedly appear. Consider the more than one billion cells that comprise our physical bodies. This unimaginable number arises predictably, yet without explanation, from one single cell after only fifty replications into 250 different types of cells. Each of these cells performs several million functions per second with no obvious instruction or apparent intervention.

No less amazing is the body's response to everything and anything. If a finger is cut, emergency response teams rush in to manage the crisis. If any form of cardiovascular activity is engaged, a symphony of synchronized activities occurs in response. The heart beats faster and pumps more blood. The lungs breathe faster and harder, blood sugar levels are elevated, conversion to carbon dioxide and water intensifies as oxygen consumption increases and energy demands escalate. Conversely, saturating the body with stimulants, antacids, carbonated beverages, lifeless foods, alcohol, medications, and numerous other poisons can directly challenge this biochemical environment. Similarly, depriving the body of sleep, subjecting it to stresses, or abusing it in untold ways, causes predictable reactions to occur.

However, directing the body's ability to respond does not coincide with creating or controlling the actual nature of the responses. The autonomic, or automatic, aspect of the nervous system governs these replies. Its counterpart, the voluntary nervous system, enacts the choices we make.

Therefore, actions can be chosen that will employ both aspects of the nervous system, but conscious control can only be asserted over one part of the interaction via the voluntary nervous system. In other words, a decision can be made to have an alcoholic beverage. This engages the voluntary nervous system to perform all related activities. Further choices can be made to frequently repeat the behavior, knowing full well what the response of the body will be. But conscious control over the automatic activities producing the response cannot be exerted.

Thus, both the body and the related biochemistry maintain intrinsic self-rule, while exhibiting a paradoxical relationship to cause and effect. "When you choose the behavior, you choose the consequences" has been popularized by television's pop psychology icon, Dr. Phil. Certainly, this holds true for the net effect it will have on the physical experience of the body. Less obvious, but no less dramatic, is the potential response it will produce in other aspects of life. Repeating a behavior causes ripples to emerge in other realms. These potential responses are far less predictable as they involve other people and their dynamics. Taken to an extreme, repeatedly choosing a socially unacceptable behavior can alter and destroy lives and relationships. What is done occasionally is not as important as what is done most of the time. Indulging occasionally is certainly not a recipe for disaster, but habitual behavior based upon repetitive choices produces a net result in the form of recurrent experiences.

Given these observations, no one knows how all of this happens. Nor is it understood how all of these functions are coordinated. On one hand, the mechanisms of many of the body's functions have been identified. These include things such as action potentials, chemical discharges, nerve impulses, neurotransmitters, receptor sites, and the like. But we have yet to identify the causal factors that trigger these behaviors and result in the transformation of our biochemistry.

Nowhere is this more obvious than in the activity of modern pharmaceuticals inside the human body. Each chemical substance comprising these wonder drugs recognizably produces far more unpredictable and undesirable side effects than desired effects. These can occur unsurprisingly in an individual experiencing a particular symptom. Of course, this occurs because anything can cause anything. The symptoms one individual may experience are not necessarily rooted in the same realm as that of another with the same symptoms. Therefore, basing treatment protocols exclusively on the presence of any particular group of symptoms results in a highly unproductive attempt to resolve a condition.

■ The Third Caveat: Everything Works

This leads to yet another caveat: "Everything works." Since there is a reaction for every action that is not necessarily an equal and opposite reaction, not everything works for everybody. Nor does every action produce the same reaction. Everything works most effectively when it is applied to a specific set of circumstances for which it is most indicated. For instance, antibiotics work well in general, but they may not be appropriate for symptoms of a cold. Nor will they necessarily be effective against all bacteria, or for all people with bacterial infections. All too often, I have seen individuals with cold-like symptoms, not linked to a germ-specific cause, prescribed a broad-spectrum antibiotic only to become worse. So too, I have seen patients with what appeared to be similar infections completely improve in response to something as simple as oil of oregano or a broad-spectrum probiotic. The same non-specific responses are seen for virtually every pharmaceutical, exercise program, diet, and stress management technique currently available.

So, despite the fact that biochemistry conforms to a somewhat linear model of observation and function (that of cause and effect), it remains a transitional arena linking the physical with the unseen realms. This relationship demonstrates an unpredictable and seemingly random pattern of behavior. As a result, part of this realm is observable and explainable, while the other is still a mystery rooted in yet another realm—that of the unseen.

The best information currently available suggests that genetics, environment and stress dictate quality of life. However from a quantum point of view, genetics merely represent a tentative expression of potential, while stress is manageable and environment is changeable. But how does this happen? What is the mechanism by which something not seen becomes something seen? Is this a totally random phenomenon, or is there some way of consciously and deliberately participating in the process?

While answers continued to emerge in response to my questions, even more questions surfaced. Is it possible that this unseen realm is actually the cause of all causes? Does whatever is going on in this realm dictate physical and/or physiological experiences? Is this a one-way street from the unseen to the seen, or does it work both ways? Is there a way to consciously access this realm and direct the energy into predictable experiences?

■ The Fourth Caveat: There Are No Panaceas

Inquiries, such as those noted above, provided the basis for discovering the factors that cause and contribute to imbalances in all three realms. The remainder of the caveats began to emerge as a manner of understanding the influences of the causes producing the effects. The caveats acquired to date served as inspiration for further exploration. Additional characteristics continued to emerge that further illustrate the paradoxical nature of this quest. The next series of insights spawned the opinion that there is no universal remedy, no panacea, and no magic potion.

This caveat is directly related to the one that precedes it, but more clearly defines the need to understand the cause when attempting to resolve a symptom complex. It also clearly demonstrates the dilemma associated with attempts to remedy healthcare concerns utilizing symptoms as the exclusive determining factor in selecting an approach to treatment.

Since anything can cause anything and everything works, the ultimate challenge is in opting for an action that produces a reaction specific to the cause of the problem. Then, and only then, can a cure be achieved, which in no way qualifies as a panacea for other like-symptoms. In the absence of a cause-specific cure, the best that can be achieved, in terms of resolving healthcare problems, is the successful result of relieving or improving symptoms through the application of substances or procedures that have consistently demonstrated an effective outcome in a given situation.

■ The Fifth Caveat: When All You Have Is a Hammer, Everything Looks Like a Nail

In addition to the caveats listed above, I have come to understand that the areas of expertise in the healing arts, referred to as specialties, are merely arenas of extensive information about a distinct feature of mortal existence. Hence the emergence of the next caveat: "When all you have is a hammer, everything looks like a nail." In other words, when something is always looked at the same way, it always looks the same.

This caveat accounts for the vast range of opinions available in response to questions about why someone is experiencing what they are experiencing. Each area of specialization in the healing arts has a distinctive rationale associated with it. Opinions regarding the cause and course of treatment for any given healthcare concern will vary according to the bias related to the particular discipline of the healthcare professional from whom you seek advice.

For example, a person with back pain will have a surplus of advice to choose from depending upon whom they consult for guidance. Every discipline has an intrinsic belief system associated with their approach to any given set of symptoms. The recommendations for managing back pain will be very different depending upon whom is consulted. A podiatrist sees the feet as the cause. A massage therapist sees the muscles as the source of the pain. A neurologist sees nerves, an orthopedic surgeon sees the spine, a neurosurgeon sees the structures inside the spine, a chiropractor sees the vertebrae, a psychologist sees the emotions, and a psychiatrist sees the mind. While these all potentially play a role in contributing to the symptoms of back pain, the inevitable cause may be somewhere entirely unrelated. If it was all as simple as one cause/one cure, there would be far fewer health care professionals and far less back pain.

Despite my best efforts to make sense of this entire process, I recognized that I must expand my diagnostic skills to include the caveats as part of my approach to differential diagnosis. In reviewing my own beliefs, experiences, training, knowledge, and expertise, I realized that they all belonged to somebody else. That is to say, I was simply accessing and regurgitating information that I had committed to memory. I reacted in a sort of knee-jerk response to a patient's stated dilemma. I was doing what I was trained to do. I was thinking someone else's thoughts and acting out the related behavior. All I had was a hammer, and everything looked like a nail.

This presented an especially burdensome predicament for me, particularly when an individual with a well-documented, previously diagnosed and chronic condition would come to me for advice, guidance, and help. Obviously they were experiencing what they were experiencing. Moreover, the diagnosis and treatments had been performed according to traditional standards. Their entire encounter had been classically contrived and constructed. Conventional teachings, beliefs, and dogma dictated the opinions they received, but without resolution. So they continued to have their experiences. But what in the world did I have to offer them?

■ The Sixth Caveat: When You Hear Hoof Beats, Look for Horses

Guided by these concerns, the challenge now became to develop a method for identifying dysfunction, impairment, imbalance, and deficiency, rather than a diagnosable disease. In so doing, I took some time to examine the progression of thought that had brought me to this crossroad. This humbling task gave me pause to reconsider my involvement in such an undertaking. Was any of this possible, or was I just a renegade idealist with a loose canon aimed at the timeless protocols of convention? How would I approach this ambiguous impediment? Where would I start?

Thank God for the wisdom of hindsight! This final question, "Where would I start?" formed the basis for launching my approach. It also contributed to a future appreciation of a related concept, "Whatever is given attention becomes more apparent," and/or "Whatever is resisted persists." Keep in mind that resistance is a form of attention that causes the object of attention to proliferate. Thus, another caveat materialized: "When you hear hoof beats, look for horses." In other words, start where you are, and look where you want to go. Between here and there is the next step in the process. Fundamentally, this is the initial step in the process of classical differential diagnosis. Unfortunately, it traditionally leads you through a conventional thought process that simply guides you to a list of the most probable diagnoses, as opposed to one of the most likely causes of the symptoms.

This caveat suggests that when a patient is experiencing a physical symptom, a physical examination is indicated as the initial effort in establishing the source of their concerns. But once again, it stops there. The goal of this conventional assessment is to identify a structure that is tentatively associated with the experience of the physical symptoms, resulting in a physical diagnosis. Conversely, the use of the hoof beats caveat merely represents a starting point for ruling out potential causes and serves as a compass for guiding one through the maze of probabilities. With the other caveats as tools for refining a direction, the ultimate destination may reside in an entirely different realm than the one in which the symptoms exist.

Before these caveats became a formal part of my routine evaluation, a paradigm shift occurred that would forever alter the way I approached these seemingly unsolvable mysteries. The paradigm shift occurred when I decided to look at these concerns in a different way. This led me to the first step of integrating the caveats into a new understanding and approach.

The first step was simply a realization. The realization was, "When you change the way you look at things, the things you look at change." I had heard self-help "guru" Wayne Dyer say this many times. But this time it really made an impact. I immediately recognized that I was onto something, but I had no idea what it was. So I began to look at things differently. I began to think for myself, perhaps for the first time since before grade school.

Nevertheless, there were still unanswered questions. Why do some things work for some people and not for others? Why do some conditions simply improve or disappear? Why does nothing ever work for some people, and/or even make their situation worse? No matter how much I knew, or how many seminars I went to, or how many techniques I learned, there was always something missing. There had to be more. And there was!

■ The Seventh Caveat: Everything Is What It Isn't

The practice of homeopathy is the therapeutic embodiment of the "everything is what it isn't" concept. It was practiced as mainstream medicine throughout the early nineteenth century. This system of healing utilizes minuscule dosages of otherwise potentially toxic substances as the basis for hastening a cure. A material that in excess would cause a disease actually becomes a remedy in therapeutic dosages. And so it is both a cause and a cure. It is what it isn't.

When coupled with the realization that when you change the way you look at things the things you look at change, everything in the visible universe becomes suspect. Integrating this fact with the other caveats provides us with a tangible model for evaluating any situation or circumstance, as well as any condition or symptom. This model offers the opportunity for us to make sense out of the unresolved issues that continue to plague us. It gives us a means for understanding the otherwise mysterious events seemingly strewn together randomly that we experience as life. It suggests an explanation as to why the perception of an encounter is often very different from what is encountered. And for me, it provided the framework for engaging the outwardly unsolvable healthcare concerns of a population frustrated with unanswered questions about their relentless symptoms.

As this process continued to unfold, it became statistically obvious that these unresolved issues were being experienced by approximately 20 percent of my patient population. Therefore, I decided to throw away the book on these individuals and begin the process of exploring what they all had in common. What they all had in common were symptoms. They were being plagued by unresolved symptoms, symptoms of imbalance, dysfunction, and deficiency. If what these unresolved cases had in common were symptoms and these symptoms were simply the effects of an underlying cause, then the obvious next step in the process was to develop an approach for identifying the cause that produced the effect. Armed with this insight and my newly acquired caveats, I proceeded to re-examine this population in the context of my new awareness.

In the process of cultivating my new awareness, more revelations appeared. Is it possible that these seemingly illusive symptoms were merely an attempt on the part of the body to communicate distress? What if these effects, which were displayed as vague symptoms, had been erroneously identified and mislabeled as "end-game" disease processes? What if these indistinct expressions of an organism in trouble are not specifically related to an identifiable "cause"? Could they simply represent the outcry of a process beginning to accumulate and develop momentum? Left unrecognized and unidentified, is it possible that these processes could eventually lead to a more familiar entity known as a diagnosable disease?

The first step must be to isolate the cause of an effect to one of the three realms, or to a dysfunction between the realms. To isolate the cause, I realized I would have to modify my approach to a common healthcare practice known as differential diagnosis. This would include some unconventional perspectives and assessments. Differential diagnosis is a systematic process of establishing a prioritized list of the most

The Seven Caveats

- Anything can cause anything.
- For every action, there is a reaction.
- Everything works.
- There are no panaceas.
- When all you have is a hammer, everything looks like a nail.
- When you hear hoof beats, look for horses.
- Everything is what it isn't.

likely names that describe an individual's experience. Most times, it is simply based upon a common group of symptoms. At times, it is remotely related to the cause. My new approach would somehow have to incorporate a consideration of cause.

■ Below the Radar

With the caveats in hand, I began to assertively explore the world of chronic and non-responsive disorders. I would eventually assign these ailments to the jurisdiction of Vicious Cycle Disorders. The population experiencing VCD consists of people with disparities more commonly referred to as sub-clinical disorders. This simply means that the source of the symptoms exists below the radar of conventional inspection. For this reason, the cause of the concerns is less than apparent and most times unobservable.

The symptoms associated with these disruptions are traditionally labeled "idiopathic," or of unknown origin. This means you have the symptoms, but we don't know where they came from, or why you have them. Nonetheless, they exist; they are real, but they evade uncomplicated recognition by concealing themselves as vague indications that something is wrong.

Most often, these patients are told that all their tests are normal, there is nothing wrong that can be seen, let's just wait and watch, or it's all in your head. Frequently, they are told that nothing is wrong, but they instinctively know that something isn't right. To accurately assess and evaluate the potential causes of their agitation, more caveats would have to emerge. And with the caveats, more familiarity, more knowledge, more perception, more awareness, more recognition, understanding, discernment, and appreciation would also have to emerge.

■ Journey through the Realms

On this journey through the realms, the above-mentioned caveats will be examined. Their application to the underlying discrepancies associated with VCD will also be explored. In addition, an investigation into the solutions for these unresolved symptoms of imbalance and dysfunction will be undertaken. A closer look at how each realm operates will then be followed by a consideration as to how each realm evolves and how it interacts with the other realms. Finally, an approach to resolving these concerns will be constructed within the context of a *Quantum Lifestyle Dynamic.*

In becoming more aware of the environment around you, you will begin to realize the promise of unlimited potential. You will then begin to consciously contribute to the development of a foundation for remodeling reality one thought at a time. These are a few of the creative processes yet to be investigated on this journey beyond the frontiers of what we think we know. In the pages that follow, the human predicament will be viewed through an assortment of eyes.

■ CHAPTER TWO ■

Vicious Cycle Disorders

"Happiness is an imaginary condition, formerly attributed by the living to the dead, now usually attributed by adults to children, and by children to adults."

—THOMAS SZASZ, THE SECOND SIN (1973) "EMOTIONS"

S ymptoms act as catalysts, hastening a desire to enter a path of practice, or to move to a different phase of your life journey. Symptoms may show you where you need to focus your attention. By seeing how much you are living in the past, you discover the importance of living in the present. By understanding the targets of your greed, you can redirect your attention to that for which you are grateful. By noticing how cynical you have become, you recognize your longing for meaning. Your symptoms equate to what you need to work on and what you desire. They are stepping-stones directly into the virtual realm. However, they can also be stumbling blocks to success if you fall prey to the pandering of the false prophets of hope promising a quick solution to your problems and contributing to the unsuspected formation of a Vicious Cycle Disorder. With the unknown still ahead, one still has to wonder what is really known about what we experience as life? People are getting sick and getting well all of the time. Mostly, no one knows why. Perhaps a part of the answer lies in the swamp of Vicious Cycle Disorders. Well, it has to be passed on the way to your new life, so why not take a quick look now?

■ How Did I Get Here?

Do you often wonder how you came to find yourself suffering from something you contributed to creating? It is not uncommon for patients to call me with concerns represented by an assortment of seemingly unrelated symptoms that constantly plague them. With no pre-established diagnosis assigned, I call these complex presentations Vicious Cycle Disorders.

A Vicious Cycle Disorder is a recurrent pattern of events that you have created. It is a continual occurrence that is experienced as some form of discontent. It is generally something that constantly nags you through the appearance of a physical or emotional complaint. It can be associated with depression, regret, remorse, unhappiness, anger, insecurity, or lack of fulfillment. Ultimately it is created by the choices that you make. The choices that you make are based upon the thoughts that you routinely entertain. These thoughts are produced by your past experiences, fears, hopes, dreams, desires, beliefs, and exposure to external stimuli.

On a practical level, it's easy to see how this might be related to adopted behaviors accumulated during the course of a lifetime. Fundamentally, if something produces a pleasurable experience, we will want to repeat it. If it produces a painful or undesirable experience, we will seek to avoid it. In essence, something is derived in the form of a tangible experience from every thought we entertain. This, in effect, is the foundation for all repetitive behavior. Repetitive behaviors gone awry account for Vicious Cycle Disorders.

While the ultimate goal is to determine the cause of these unrelenting burdens, it is equally important to understand how they develop. One of the benefits and curses of "free will" is that we get to choose our actions. Action creates memory and memory creates desire, which leads back again to action. Thus, the designation of a Vicious Cycle Disorder. Oftentimes, these vague symptoms are related to lifestyle choices and behaviors. Frequently, it is forgotten that when a behavior is chosen, so too are the consequences. As a result, self-created suffering is difficult to distinguish.

Developing awareness becomes critical to resolving these types of complaints. Incorporating some type of daily practice to cultivate this awareness is as important as any other aspect of a well-rounded wellness program. Spiritual practices exist in all traditions and cultures. The techniques are different, but the goal is the same: to calm the mind and facilitate the integration of the realms. These practices can include any style of discipline that accomplishes these purposes. Examples of these rituals can include yoga, meditation, tai chi, postures, breathing exercises, chanting, prayers, exercise and diet. All too frequently, most problems are approached exclusively through the physical or biochemical realms, while neglecting the virtual realm altogether.

■ Quantum Insights

While highly technical at first glance, no discussion of the virtual would be complete without at least a passing mention of the interpretations offered by a bizarre world of organized chaos known as quantum physics. Aside from the disciplined structures used to communicate the essence of this seemingly unintelligible branch of science, quantum physics offers insight into the dynamics of Vicious Cycle Disorders. It does this through the eyes of a concept called wave-particle duality that forms the basis of modern thought relative to our existence and potential as human beings. With one foot in the swamp of Vicious Cycle Disorders, the other is free to dip into the lake of subatomic particles comprising the virtual realm.

To give you some perspective on this short course of quantum phenomenon and its relationship to the subject matter of this book, simply understand that physics is essentially concerned with the way matter interacts with other matter. Quantum physics is just the physics of the incredibly small. It attempts to explain the behavior of these very, very small particles. The reason that quantum physics needs complex math to explain these behaviors and properties is because the world of subatomic particles is filled with probabilities and organized chaos. While you don't have to understand these concepts to consciously change your life experience, it can be helpful to understand that there are some distinct principles that govern activities, and which influence the results of the choices you make to create your life experiences. You can consciously employ these principles to achieve any desired result.

■ Physics, Meaning, and Consciousness

Although this makes for fascinating reading, it's a bit much for what we want to accomplish right now. You're probably wondering, what does any of this have to do with anything? Physics has in this century begun invading the realm of meaning and consciousness. Contemporary physics guru Gary Zukav, in a recent history of physics, explains that John Von Neumann's "discovery that our thought processes (the realm of symbols) project illusory restrictions onto the real world leads to essentially the same discovery that led Einstein to the general theory of relativity."

The general theory of relativity shows us that the human mind follows different rules than the real world does. A rational mind, with the impressions that it receives from its limited perspective, forms structures that thereafter determine what it further will and will not freely accept. From that point on, regardless of how the real world actually operates, this rational mind follows its own self-imposed rules and tries to superimpose on the real world its own version of what must be. Taking a closer look at subatomic particles as a group, the behaviors known as Vicious Cycle Disorders can then be defined. Simply put, the best way to define the future is to create it. From the library of ancient Egypt's Alexandria comes this paraphrased reassurance. The universe is wholly connected. It includes us and responds to our every whim. It allows for us to define our vision and make adjustments as we collect data. Our thoughts define what is and what is to be, while our feelings and emotions provide the impetus for manifesting a desired reality.

In the chapter dealing with the biochemical realm, we will see how small particles, such as neuropeptides, molecules, and receptors, participate in creating our life experiences as part of a second nervous system fluid enough to match the activities of the mind. Although these substances are not thoughts, they move like thoughts, serving as transformers between the mind and the body. These seemingly unconnected entities of thoughts and bodily reactions are intimately related. Transformations of the nonmatter thoughts manifest themselves as our physical experiences. Similarly, the use and interpretation of language serves as a tangible expression of thought processes that mimic the effects illustrated by the shadows emerging on a wall from an invisible light source. These transformations are also within the conscious control of focused efforts we can learn to employ.

■ Subatomic States

Earlier, I mentioned a concept called wave-particle duality. Further study reveals that all subatomic particles exist in two states. The first is a particle. Particles have been thought to be the building blocks of all the solid objects in our world. The other subatomic state is that of a wave. Waves were originally believed to be nonsolid, such as sound and light waves. At the time this concept was proposed, there was believed to be no overlap. Particles were particles and waves were waves. Ultimately, it was determined that both were both, but neither was neither until it was observed. The importance of this scientific finding relative to our participation in the creation of VCD is simply that nothing exists until it is observed. In other words, we contribute to the creation of our own personal reality by paying attention to something.

■ Hazy Thoughts

As a consequence, the hazy-wave exists as potential for a behavior to exist in the form of a thought. This means that anything is possible, but it becomes more probable if it is given attention. The more attention something is given, the more likely it will exist as part of the reality we create for ourselves. Subsequently, without the consciousness of the virtual realm to initiate observation, every thought exists only as a potential event. Once we decide to act on the vague concept of a thought, it becomes a reality. Repeatedly attending to the same process of thought produces the habitual behavior of attending to the same process

The Point of It All

- We each have approximately 60,000 thoughts per day.
- These thoughts exist as possibilities until we assign attention to them, i.e. choose to observe them.
- Once observed (or chosen), the probability that they will reoccur is increased.
- The action of choosing a possibility is based upon our genetics, environment, and exposure to stress.
- Choosing a possibility creates a memory.
- The memory serves as a catalyst, creating a desire for repeating or avoiding the choice.

of thought. That process subsequently produces a tangible result in our physical experience of reality.

So lives are made real by acting on the infinite number of possible choices available, thus creating a memory of that experience and the potential for repeating it. If it produced a pleasurable result, the desire to experience it again is produced. Thus, patterns of behavior emerge, and the choices we make most frequently determine how we got where we are at any one point. This repeated action of thinking the same thoughts increases the probability that these thoughts and behaviors will occur again.

Everyone strives for a sense of wholeness and purpose in life. Our true nature is to be complete and at one with the divine. Somewhere along our path, it seems we have lost our way. We have become fragmented and cut off from truth. We no longer feel that we have control over our lives. We all engage in destructive patterns of behavior that keep us from our true sense of power. This, in turn, produces the fear spoken of by Nelson Mandela when he suggested that our greatest fear is not that we are powerless, but that we are far more powerful than we think.

The learned responses we have adopted to cope with what was being done or said to us at a certain time are not who we really are. Life is a quest to be whole. Disease is rooted in the belief that we are incomplete. Our spiritual journey, then, is to work at becoming whole by reconnecting with all those pieces that we have denied, disowned, or otherwise suppressed.

■ The Influence of Behavior

Since nothing is intrinsically good or bad, but dependent upon a relative perspective, the net effect of behavior is dependent upon the context within which it is experienced. However, certain behaviors do have inherent qualities and characteristics that dictate some general consequences. The theoretical influence of common behaviors can be studied in the following examples involving all three realms.

Take something as simple as the execution of routine daily functions. You awaken from sleep and perform your morning rituals. Regardless of what it involves, it is a habit you've chosen and acquired. This ritual is a pattern of behavior that you have adopted based upon your training, exposure, desires, and choices. Good, bad or indifferent, this ritual consists of the basic elements you have incorporated to prepare you for the day you are about to begin. From the moment you arise, the thoughts you entertain and the activities in which you participate exemplify the reward/avoidance system that characterizes the inspiration for embracing the experiences you are about to encounter.

Even the mundane tasks of showering, shaving, primping, dressing, and preparing to depart are adopted patterns which will order the environment in which you will experience your life on any given day. Expanded to include some of our less obvious penchants, patterns of behavior surface as relatively common activities. For instance, downtime is Americans' favorite pastime. We zone out with television, radio, the Internet, shopping, parties, movies, hanging out, and working out. Some equate to bad habits, some are therapy, but most are escapes from the routines of daily life.

■ Is This All There Is?

Upon closer inspection, we begin to ask, is this all there is? These routine blueprints that form the labyrinth of life are seemingly harmless habits like watching too much television, over-shopping, surfing the Internet, talking on the phone, or things we overdo without realizing it. It seems like normal behavior because we do it repeatedly. Besides, everyone else is doing it, too. Depending upon the nature, frequency, and purpose of these habits, they may be a problem if they are used as an escape from a life of conscious choices.

It's true! Anything in excess can be problematic. So you need to ask yourself: "How excessive is it, and how much does it interfere with my ability to consciously construct the life I really want to live?" Not all mindless indulgences are bad habits. There's a place in our lives for pointless conversations, reruns of *Friends*, and double chocolate fudge swirl. To some extent, we do these things to cope with the stress in our lives. It's legitimate after a stressful day to take some time to vegetate. The significance lies in what we choose to do, how we choose to do it, and how frequently we engage in it. The solutions we employ will determine the ultimate consequences.

■ Choosing Behavior

The frequency and consistency with which you engage in a particular behavior is far less a determining factor in shaping consequence than what behavior you choose. When you're overworked, addicted to caffeine, sugar, or alcohol, then there may be consequences in your physical and mental acuity. Subsequent behavioral choices may lead you to seek relief from these stressful feelings and persuade you to calm down by sitting in front of the tube with a TV dinner, your favorite beer, and stay up too late. If you're tired the next day and engage in a similar scenario, this could be the beginning of a Vicious Cycle Disorder. If that's all you do, and you do it every night and every weekend, it becomes woven into the fabric of a behavior pattern that contributes to the propagation of VCD. Habitually just going through the motions becomes a problem. These habits keep us from living a life of greater meaning and experiencing the satisfaction that we really want and deserve. They focus our attention on experiences that prevent us from evolving. Unfortunately, the connection is usually less than obvious.

Tips for Changing Your Experience

- Understand the world you live in: Study and apply the concepts offered by quantum physics to actively engage the mechanisms within your control for consciously creating. Knowing the landscape will help you to map out an approach to change and establish goals.
- Acquire and implement the tools necessary to produce the changes you desire. This will require a reallocation of your energy and focus by selecting a compatible discipline and being consistent in its application.
- Monitor your progress. Make periodic adjustments to keep you focused and headed in the direction of correction. Don't be afraid to explore. Be receptive to change.

■ Soft Addictions

Once we are aware of this behavior and the consequences, we are free to choose alternatives. Because of their subtle nature, these repetitive patterns of behavior are known as soft addictions. So, in essence, what we are really talking about here are habits. A habit is something you do repeatedly. These activities will form the memories that are a part of the 60,000 thoughts you will have each day. Good, bad, or indifferent, regardless of how you perceive your past actions, their effect on your tomorrow will be proportionate to the amount of attention you assign them. Eventually, the actual habitual activity becomes cloaked in a veil of symptoms that evolve out of the activity. At that point, your focus changes. Now you have a group of vague symptoms consuming your interest. Now the actual cause of the symptoms becomes a vague memory lost in the commotion of a Vicious Cycle Disorder.

■ Freedom to Change

Changing these soft addictions isn't easy, particularly when you remain oblivious to the underlying cause. But there are some predictable and powerful methods for attending to them. The seed of any new experience lies in awareness. Identifying the fact that they exist is the first step. This awareness causes us to focus our attention. Attention begets intention. If this intention is to change, your attention is suddenly expanded toward opportunities that will support your intention. Suddenly, the universe conspires to facilitate your purpose and an attraction polarity is established. Oftentimes, this process can be enhanced with the alteration of one simple aspect of your routine activities.

Maybe you head out shopping every Saturday morning. Next time, schedule a walk with a friend or a bicycle ride instead. This way, you've broken the routine and added something more nourishing to your life. Look for other things that you might enjoy. It accelerates the process, since nothing exists until it is observed. As your fascination for change becomes heightened, add more things to your new routine. Soon, you'll be cutting back on routine behaviors, but you won't feel deprived. This is frequently referred to as the "Math of More." You learn to add more nourishing things to your life, so you can subtract your soft addictions. Eventually, you'll come to enjoy these new things so much they crowd out your soft addictions.

■ Two Mechanisms of VCD

In the final analysis, Vicious Cycle Disorders represent symptoms of imbalance that are undetectable with conventional analysis. They are initiated by one of two mechanisms. The first is that of a habitual behavior based upon recurrent choices in any one of the three realms. The other is by something you have yet to discover until you become aware of it. Each possibility eventually becomes more probable as your exposure escalates. Each requires a different method of analysis and identification. Each of the two is associated with a particular type of magnetism that engages your attention. Each is closely aligned with a choice that serves to comfort you and make you feel more secure. This feeling of security can motivate you to pursue the experience repeatedly.

■ Techniques for Change

Meanwhile, there are several very effective techniques for facilitating a conscious relationship with behavior. A comprehensive discussion of viable options and how to choose them is presented in the chapter on Quantum Lifestyle Dynamics. But I do want to touch on one very simple and powerful technique here, called journaling. Journaling is writing out your daily thoughts, and it is a tremendous self-help instrument capable of contributing to the journey back to self.

There are some simple techniques to help you get the most out of your journaling experience. For starters, find a comfortable place to begin, clear your mind, and relax. Let your thoughts and emotions flow freely. Do not censor yourself as you write. Don't worry about grammar or punctuation. Put all of your thoughts into writing. Be yourself.

Writing helps to clarify your feelings, so first choose a topic, follow your feelings, and write. Write about something that makes you happy or sad. Write about something you've discovered. Write about your desires, your needs, your fears, and your curiosities. Try to write everyday and at the same time of day. Be consistent.

Tedious as it sounds, the benefits of journaling provide a powerful tool for creating and monitoring intentions. It can provide tremendous insight into the so-called problem areas of your life by focusing your attention and allowing you to look at things differently. There's something magical about taking time to write down a bigger vision for your life. With this process, your new choices have a context. They begin to make sense in terms of your priorities. It's not a quick fix, nor is it going to happen overnight, but it's part of the process of consciously creating the life you actually want to live. It's really about learning to live the journey of life. And it's cumulative. Once you've developed momentum, you're on your way to discovering who you really are and being where you want to be. An ancient Chinese proverb states that, "Unless we change direction, we are likely to end up where we are headed."

■ Symptom Solutions

With the caveats as your guides, you have some effective tools for sorting out the differential diagnosis of your own lives. For example, if you're feeling stressed, you can seek a remedy by responding to a commercial solicitation promising resolution of the symptoms through a pill that suppresses the production of cortisol. You could also choose to stop for a moment and listen to the sounds of hoof beats, which suggest that the stresses producing the excess cortisol need to be identified, minimized, eliminated, managed, or reorganized.

If you are dealing with the symptom of excess weight, you could hop on the merry-go-round of pills and diets designed to produce "incredible results" and produce additional issues for you to deal with at a later date. You could also stop for a minute to recognize that there are no panaceas, and that everything works. You could then initiate a search for a process that will allow you to identify the behaviors and beliefs that are contributing to relentless symptoms and seek a solution specific to your needs. If you are dealing with the symptoms of a physiological dysfunction causing high cholesterol, high blood pressure, hot flashes, headaches, or skin rashes, there's a pill for that. But there's also a solution, if you look in the right place.

■ Looking in the Right Place

Perhaps we are looking for answers in all the wrong places. Perhaps we assume that if something manifests itself as a physical ailment, the cause must be rooted in the physical realm as well. Since there are three realms, statistically there is a one-third possibility of this being true. In fact, in many of the cases I've evaluated, an unexpected trauma, nutritional deficiencies or chronic imbalances are at the root of the associated physical problems. But this is the benefit of having the caveats to serve as guides. In a symptom complex associated with a physical cause, when you hear hoof beats, you find horses. However, when what appears to be obvious does not respond to the obvious, then the cause typically resides in one of the other two realms.

If the physical symptoms seem to have no causal basis in the physical realm, then because of the dynamic process of realm interaction, the biochemical realm is explored next. If the treatment directed toward the biochemical realm does not improve the physical symptoms, then the virtual realm must be evaluated next.

If you are dealing with depression, anxiety, insomnia, unhappiness, lack of self-esteem, anger, frustration, lack of fulfillment, or any other intangible symptom of affliction, you could "ask your doctor," or you could "ask yourself." At some point, you must recognize and acknowledge that relief is not necessarily a long-term answer. You must also submit to the fact that life and its experiences are a process. Consequently, it is by your conscious or unconscious participation that circumstances, situations, and symptoms arise.

■ The Source of Symptoms

Ultimately, you are always nearer to the source of your symptoms than any outside reference because you are the source of your own experiences. As you sift your encounters through the filters of perception, you alone become responsible for the consequences, the results, the responses, and the symptoms. While superficially this may sound harsh, unrealistic, and impractical, it is also full of promise and hope. As you begin to accept responsibility for your actions, you also assume influence over the reactions. Thus, you begin to move from the domain of physical encounters, through the conduit of biochemical transformation, and on to the virtual realm.

The emptiness, loneliness, and dissatisfaction you feel along your journey through the more tangible realms will be more than compensated for by your arrival in the virtual. After all, the expression of symptoms in the other realms is a mere reflection of our discontent in our virtual realm. In feeling that you have lost contact with your creative origins, you frantically seek to fill the developing void with indulgences. This provides little more than temporary gratification, which proves fleeting at best. These transitory efforts to restore a sense of wholeness fall short of your true aspirations. With each failed attempt to satisfy your desires, you become more vulnerable to the promises of predators seeking to realize their own visions through your quiet desperation.

■ Personal Agendas

You probably have your own reasons for wanting to start this journey. Perhaps you have experienced some kind of awakening and know that your life will never be the same. If you were raised in one of the world's religions, you may have come to a point where you want to further dip into the spiritual river. Perhaps you suspect that there's something more to life, or you're just curious. But most of us are drawn to the virtual realm because, as a doctor might say, certain symptoms are "presenting."

You might feel that something is missing in your life, something you desperately want. You could be longing for inspiration, or community, or quality time. You could be in pain and in need of healing. You could be feeling happy and grateful and compelled to give something back to the universe. You could be facing a crisis and know that how you handled such situations in the past won't be enough this time. You could be burned out. You could be worried about your loved ones or frightened about the very real dangers in the world. You might be sensing that your life could be more meaningful, but you don't know how to go about making it so.

Take heart! These real-life feelings, challenges, and experiences are just what the journey into the virtual realm is all about. I like to call them *practices for human being* because they are being done in the midst of your life. Defined simply, virtual disciplines are practices or activities performed in an effort to move into a deeper and more meaningful relationship with your true self, other people, or the whole of creation.

On the path to our final destination of the unseen realm, some amazing facts and bewildering oddities will be encountered. By now, all of your conventional senses are heightened. You're beginning to learn how to look at things in different ways and see things you didn't know existed. The way you hear, smell, touch, taste, and observe will all be enhanced by default. What's more, you've begun to recognize that there are things to experience and ways of experiencing them that you never imagined. In the words of Albert Einstein, "Imagination is more important than knowledge." Your curiosity has been stirred and your awareness energized. But, you're not quite there yet. There are still things to learn that will help to bring your excursion into focus as you move toward integrating your wisdom into a workable model for living.

■ Perceptual Reality

Given that you experience the physical world through your senses of sight, sound, taste, touch, and smell, much of what goes on in the physical universe remains unattainable due to the finite capabilities of these conduits. Your eyes are sensitive only to a narrow range of frequencies that precludes visual access to the fields of infrared, microwaves, radio waves, X-rays, and gamma rays. So visually, your perceptions leave you privy to only a small portion of what is actually there.

The other senses provide a similarly limited capacity. The ears perceive only the range of sound frequencies they are genetically attuned to distinguish. Moreover, there is no real sound in the world of material reality. There are simply waves of pressure, which exert an influence on the instruments of interpretation. And so it goes with all of your senses. The physical realities of electromagnetic fields, lingering scents, polarized light, sonar waves, and electrical fields, all elude the awareness of the human senses. Stop for a moment to observe all of the things you are unaccustomed to being aware of. A new and heightened sense of awareness begins to emerge.

■ Becoming Aware

As you consciously encourage yourself to become more aware, you are led to the brink of the virtual realm. This is where you begin to recognize that the entire world of your experience is a manifestation within your own mind. It is at this point that you can initiate a new journey undefined by boundaries. From this vantage point, you can begin to see what your eye has not seen and hear what your ear has not heard. Hence, you can embark on a journey of observation predicated not by the senses alone, but upon the potential that exists as a fundamental component of consciousness.

It is now time to observe the events of your daily lives through the eye, which does not see, and the ear, which does not hear. As Ralph Waldo Emerson put it, "People only see what they are prepared to see." If I look through your eyes, will I see as you see, or will I simply see myself through your eyes? To adequately answer this question, the anatomy of the virtual realm must be dissected. The relationship of this realm to the others must also be dissected. As St. Augustine said, "People travel to wonder at the height of the huge waves of the sea, at the long courses of rivers, at the vast compass of the ocean, at the circular motion of the stars; and they pass by themselves without wondering."

■ The Springboards of Limitation

Peering into the relationship of the realms, a phrase from *The Cloud of Unknowing* hints of the voyage before us: "a nature found within all creatures but not restricted to them; outside all creatures, but not excluded from them." Know that the limited dimensions in which we interact with the physical world by no means designate the limitations of our experience. Rather than representing a finite boundary, limitations can serve as a springboard from which we may choose to engage the infinite potential of purpose.

From here, you may acknowledge through direct personal experience that your entire world is a manifestation within the mind. Realize that it is the world in you and not you in the world. As this new paradigm takes seed, you begin to bear the fruit of conscious participation in your own process. You may then begin to take responsibility for your life by monitoring what you think and how you respond to any encounter. Recall that your ability to consciously participate in the creation of your daily encounters is predicated upon your genetics, the environment in which you developed, and the character of stress you regularly negotiate. It's easy to see how the capacity for evolving may vary. It is within the framework of your early evolution on this planet that you cultivate the mechanisms for functioning in your environment. During the first several years following birth, you are exposed to attitudes, opinions, prejudices, beliefs, behaviors and experiences. These inevitably dictate the operating system you will subscribe to in dealing with experiences you encounter as you mature.

For many, these early occurrences will define a life-long quest for self-worth and meaning. For others, these initial exposures will serve as the motivation to question the status quo and pursue alternatives. In either event, the expressed potential is defined by curiosity, receptivity, and, to some extent, the level of dissatisfaction experienced. Success in achieving fulfillment is predicated upon adopted belief systems and the awareness developed as a result of motivation, persistence, and discipline.

■ A Thorough Self-Examination

By this time, the multidimensional nature of the human experience is well established. Life is encountered on a daily basis through contact with all of these dimensions to varying degrees, depending upon where your attention is concentrated. If you have been conditioned to expect struggle, problems, difficulties, and unhappiness, then your attention to these potential occurrences will polarize the convergence of similar events into high probabilities of recurrence. These probabilities will be enhanced by your exposure to influences that reinforce the likelihood of repetition. This repetition is at the heart of VCD.

This scenario can be exemplified by someone who has been habituated to always expect the "other shoe to drop," regardless of the pleasantness of any recent experience. To minimize these effects, one must begin to establish an objective perspective regarding his or her basic conditioning. Starting from where you are will ensure that where you go next will not be dictated by where you have been.

A thorough self-examination at this point will be of tremendous value prior to immersing yourself in the virtual realm. Simply being aware of what you do and how you do it will contribute tremendously to your ability to make other choices more consciously. Being frustrated by what you are experiencing in your life is entirely different than recognizing that you are frustrated with what you have created. Keep in mind that there is a huge difference between taking responsibility for your choices and blaming yourself or others for what you have chosen.

■ Critical Choices

It is at this crossroads that choices become critical to your eventual fate. Embracing your responsibility provides the foundation for returning to a healthy relationship with yourself. Avoiding this opportunity to reconnect with yourself often leads to choices that reunite you with destructive behavior. These usually present themselves in the form of negative thoughts, words, desires, and actions.

In some manner, the choices you make out of frustration are embedded in a deep desire for fulfillment. Many times, you simply lose your way, mistaking the short-lived pleasure of indulgence as a true remedy for your discontentment. At times, you begin to truly believe that this destructive behavior is all there is, and so you seek more of it.

Nonetheless, eventually you come to realize that there is more. But you have no idea how to find it. And so you begin the treacherous journey inward, which is littered with the debris of accumulated past efforts. But the debris can also serve as a stepping stone to a plateau from which you can begin to observe. And as you begin to observe, you begin to see things differently. And as you look at things differently, the things you look at change. And as things change, you change. Then you realize that you have been here all along. You just didn't realize it. So you begin to make different choices. With these different choices, you begin to feel the exhilaration of co-creating a rewarding and fulfilling future as you embrace your destiny with fervor, zeal, commitment, and enthusiasm.

You begin to freely observe from a detached perspective how you have contributed to your own negative experiences in each of the three realms. In so doing, you have contributed to the creation of VCD in your own life. Embracing the operating parameters of your early life, you can scrutinize your participation in the realms. You can also monitor your development from this point forward.

■ Life Exposures

In doing this, you will no doubt recognize how your life experiences have contributed to who you are now, and how you feel about your life. Obviously, your early family life forms a large part of the foundation upon which subsequent endeavors are based. It provides you with an introduction to opinions, learned behaviors, attitudes, and prejudices. It also contributes to the many patterns of behavior that allow Vicious Cycle Disorders to emerge as dominant elements in one or more of your personal realms of existence.

The activities you are encouraged to engage in as a youth contribute to your current physical status. The behaviors you are exposed to establish the premise for your future choices. Oftentimes, these latent activities serve as precursors for VCD in a specific realm. More than frequently, an environment filled with anger, resentment, frustration, anxiety, depression, and self-deprecation serves as a springboard for an endless series of related behaviors contributing to an unfulfilled life.

Consider all of the subtle enticements you have been exposed to in the process of maturing. In the progression of your frantic individual life, it is easy to forget that everyone else has been exposed to similar events and circumstances, too. It certainly becomes all that much easier to criticize and blame when you lose sight of, or never acquire, an objective viewpoint that helps you recognize that we're all in this together.

■ Recreating Our Lives

Your individual perspective serves as a lens through which you view the world. Depending upon your focus, it is easy to get stuck in the drama of your present life circumstances. All too often, it is easier to condemn and punish, rather than learn and grow. Thus, your thoughts begin to design

Tools for Transformation

- Adopt a discipline that allows you direct access to the source of creation—your thoughts. Practice, be flexible, and be consistent.
- Recognize that the physical world is an effect, not a cause. It is the result of your thoughts, words, and actions.
- Learn to believe and expect. Understand that the only limits are those you impose upon yourself.
- Understand the laws of cause and effect. Use them to produce your desired results.
- Find your purpose and dedicate your energy to achieving it.
- Let go of things that aren't working for you. Begin by substituting behaviors that have the potential to produce what you really want.
- Constantly be aware of how your choices are producing what you experience and become congruent in your attitude, thought, words, and actions.

your destiny. They impact not just your future, but the broader future of the planet's collective consciousness as well.

Given the various elements of your upbringing, countless opportunities abound to propagate insecurity or to enhance well-being. The desire to experience the promise of unlimited potential through conscious choice intensifies as you draw closer to an exploration of the virtual realm. You may find yourself both more receptive and more anxious. It is helpful to disengage your prior conceptions and suspend any disbelief in anticipation of relearning and recreating a liberated life of endless possibilities. With your awareness heightened, it becomes easy to recognize the potential snares along the way. There are innumerable enticements that offer what you think you want in the form of something you don't really need. But as you continue to look at things differently, you can quickly distinguish what has the potential to bring you closer to the sense of self-sufficiency that you really desire.

■ CHAPTER THREE ■
Virtual Reality

"Reality is that which, when you stop believing in it, doesn't go away."
— Philip K. Dick, "Do Androids Dream of Electric Sheep?"
U.S. science fiction author (1928–1982)

The human tendency is to localize treatment of physical symptoms to the system in which they appear. It must be remembered that the physical being and biological processes are not isolated entities, but actually provide influence for the organism as a whole. Since each of the realms is merely an aspect of the same human experience, every disease has a component of each of the realms and each realm has the seeds of every disease. Differentiating between illnesses traceable to somatic causes, and those that appear to mimic them, can often be accomplished by observing the relationships between mind and body, the emotions and their expressions. Often, it is easy to be deceived by functional disturbances of the nervous system that represent a physiological interaction between the physical and virtual realms. This discrepancy in diagnosis persists because of a natural tendency to gravitate toward a more tangible reality. Often, a virtual disruption provides the foundation for the expression of related symptoms in another realm. They quickly resolve once identified and the patient is recognized to be a whole person representative of the sum of all of his or her parts. However, a functional dynamic that includes the influences of intangible origins must first be acknowledged to achieve this perspective. These influences can eventually be considered to be causal factors of the resulting imbalance.

■ Life Is a Symptom

Once the existence of an unseen realm is acknowledged, it can be helpful to remember that all of life's experiences are affected by the dynamic interaction of the three realms. In fact, life itself is a symptom that arises from the innate activity of the virtual realm. In other words, the hidden dynamic of each of the individual realms affects each of the others. It is also important to recognize that these realms are different but related aspects of the human experience. While each realm serves a distinct purpose and has unique qualities, each also shares a common evolutionary process that links one to another, making them interdependent. Therefore, the nature and extent of their interaction produces a result that we experience as our lives.

Acknowledging this reality presents an opportunity to explore new ways that can get you around any impasse in your personal experience. If you are willing to acknowledge the possibility that this realm and the dynamics I describe actually exist, then you are ready to explore the virtual realm.

Simple identification and observation are all that is needed to explore the physical and biochemical realms. These basic mechanisms provide the framework for isolating cause-and-effect relationships that operate in a predictably linear fashion. This is the basis of conventional medical assessment, differential diagnosis, and the scientific process.

Applying these tools allows an understanding of the how and why of an infinite number of phenomena that occurs repeatedly in our daily lives. The essence of this dynamic can be observed and characterized in the form of isolated interactions. This basic cause-and-effect process is reproducible and consistent. In fact, it is the foundation for our routine daily encounters, and serves as the basis for all teachable knowledge.

These predictable mechanisms also serve as a launch pad for an excursion into the void that underlies our tangible experiences. This is the virtual realm. For many, the journey into this realm is too intimidating and surreal, and, therefore, is never undertaken. Others remain curious and intrigued by the possibilities of the virtual realm, but only a few venture out into this inner world of wonder and awe.

The price of admission to the virtual realm is merely the time it takes to engage a thought. The reality of this realm is that while choosing not to actively participate in it, or not to consciously acknowledge it, everyone contributes to it. Despite its intangible nature, the tangible effects of its presence can be felt, experienced, and observed everywhere.

■ Examples of Common Imbalances

Examples of these types of imbalances might involve scenarios in which injuries are incurred in a motor vehicle accident, but trigger active symptoms in the biochemical or virtual realms. In cases of this type, the patient is usually predisposed to an expression of symptoms in one of the other two realms. Take, for example, a person who is actively dealing with a variety of concerns involving their health, long-term security, a troubled relationship or self-esteem problems. They may choose to use the precipitating accident as an opportunity to service these otherwise subclinical worries by deliberately or subconsciously exaggerating their physical concerns. Subsequently, the imbalance causing their long-term suffering is actually rooted in one realm, but triggered by an incident in a totally different realm. Often, these symptoms are so significant that it becomes difficult to recognize their true cause.

I recall one of several such incidents involving a middle-aged female who was happily married and gainfully employed. Despite some longstanding, physical imbalances involving weight gain and degenerative spinal conditions, she was always pleasant and optimistic. However, following a motor vehicle accident, she failed to respond as expected to conservative therapy. Nonetheless, she continued to receive treatment faithfully. She also continued to engage a rather large collection of healthcare professionals, who all focused on her lack of physical response.

It wasn't until years after the accident and repeated clinical encounters that she began to express her deep unhappiness and depression. In the final analysis, she disclosed a tremendous dislike for her job, concerns about her financial future, and a lack of self-esteem. Her physical ailments were obvious, legitimate and tangible. Her accident was an opportunity for her to resolve her true emotional concerns using the physical complaints as a means to an end. Almost miraculously, once this mechanism was identified and acknowledged, her physical symptoms improved to the point of merely being an infrequently spoken of inconvenience.

In a comparable scenario, another female with a similarly cheerful disposition suddenly developed a bizarre conglomeration of symptoms believed to be associated with the early onset of menopause. These symptoms appeared to emerge almost spontaneously in virtually every system of her body. Ultimately, it was discovered that these physiological symptoms were related to a deep-seated disdain for her job and her employer. She engaged a multitude of healthcare professionals in an attempt to remedy her overt physical symptoms, but to no avail. During the course of our conversations, I determined that her actual subconscious goal was to extract herself from a very stressful situation. As a result, her subconscious intention expressed itself as a mass of vague, multi-system symptoms in an attempt to influence her providers into a frenzied state of frustration sufficient enough to recommend total and permanent disability.

■ Reasonable Expectations

These stories reflect a mere sampling of actual case histories of patients that routinely arrive in my office. Most of the scenarios present themselves and unfold in a fairly similar fashion. Nonetheless, not all necessarily end the same way. Often, the presenting symptoms improve or resolve themselves with simple, accurate, focused intervention. My clinical observations over the years suggest that ninety percent of the patients achieve ninety percent of their improvement within ninety days. It is also within this time frame that primary causal factors can typically be identified, competently allocated to the appropriate realm, and dealt with in a suitable manner.

Restoring optimal function to someone experiencing symptoms rooted in biochemistry could typically take anywhere from three to six months, and in some cases up to a year. If the cause is rooted in either of the other two realms, it may take longer. If the other two realms are merely compensating for the biochemical imbalance, biochemical integrity can be achieved in as little as eight to twelve weeks.

Unfortunately, when symptoms arise from an imbalance that is firmly rooted in the virtual realm, there is no cure in either of the other two realms. When an individual suffering from an imbalance of this nature is inclined to dismiss the possibility of such a dynamic, they are doomed to suffer the consequences. As we will observe a little later, it is highly likely that all symptoms are actually rooted in the virtual realm. In other words, life is a psychosomatic experience. Simply put, this label is meant to suggest an interrelationship between the psychological (virtual) and physiological (physical) aspects of all normal and abnormal bodily functions. Thus, the human experience could be referred to as a "psychobiological event."

The mystifying territory of the unseen is a field dominated by energy and information. Everything in this realm is indistinct, vague, formless, delicate and insubstantial. This realm cannot be perceived by any of the five senses, yet it constitutes the causal foundation of everything in the observable universe. The material world is a manifestation of the unseen and the unseen comprises the source of energy from which the physical emerges.

Everything in this realm occurs beyond the speed of light. This is certainly the most dynamic realm. It is also the one with the most potential because it is a realm of pure unexpressed possibilities. It is independent from conscious physical existence, and yet mysteriously links us through the nervous system as co-conspirators by virtue of thoughts and their interpretation.

The simple act of prayer is a silent acknowledgment of a belief in this realm. The fact that some prayers appear to go unanswered contributes to confusion, disappointment, and frustration regarding the unseen realm. The frustration with the results of random requests disguised as prayers is simply that they appear to be so inconsistent. However, prayer is anything but inconsistent; it is simply misunderstood.

A response to every request is provided, but frustration exists in the failure to recognize what has really been asked for and how it's been asked. As we are reminded in the book of James, "We have not, because we ask not. We ask and receive not, because we ask amiss." So, the first and most obvious way to create the life we desire is to learn how to access the abundant storehouse of potential responses to our requests. Spiritual disciplines and practices are designed to assist us in establishing this relationship. This vast inventory is waiting to be distributed through a process of attainment commonly known as prayer. It is this process of prayer that reliably helps to provide the desired response. But there is a big difference between thinking and praying. Prayer has a direction. It is not simply focusing on the ceaseless chatter inside your head, sharing with friends, talking to a spiritual leader or venting to a psychologist. Prayer is a name for a very specific process of action and reaction initiated by you with the intention of producing the desired result in your life. So, in reality you control the outcome of this interaction by virtue of the way in which you apply the principles of operation. In the final analysis, all prayer is answered; however asking amiss produces just that, a miss.

■ The Nature of Reality

Models have been constructed to define relationships within the various versions of reality that different people have chosen to subscribe. As a result, there is a common disagreement over which is the one "true" nature of reality. Since everything is what it isn't, everyone is right and everyone is wrong. Nonetheless, the very nature of the inquiry depicts a commonality in the efforts. What is sought after is an explanation for something that can't be seen, felt, or touched with the five conventional senses. And so, in approaching a conscious interaction with the virtual realm, we must first construct a process for exploring the unknown using what we do know. The foundation for this endeavor is the same caveat we used for our differential diagnosis in the physical and biochemical realms: "When you hear hoof beats, look for horses." Awareness is a kind of "horse" that can help define the framework for a virtual encounter. It is important to note, however, that the starting point for such an exploration is arbitrary. Keep in mind that humans are the only known species capable of being aware that they are aware.

■ The Substance of Non-Substance

The virtual realm exists as a theoretical division beyond the point at which it can be detected with the five senses or any other instrument. Immersed in the journey of a collective earthly life, a realization emerges that suggests that there is something else out there. This something else must exist somewhere between what is known and what is not known.

Eventually, this theorizing leads to a place of non-substance, which in itself is the substance from which all possibilities emerge. Since everything is what it isn't, the perception of an encounter is often very different from what is encountered. Somewhere between these two interrelated phenomena is a world where an underlying reality provides for a perceptual interpretation by the senses. It is in this world that the apparent solidity of the known universe begins to disappear.

An inspection of the debris of the miraculous in each of the realms will reveal that a relationship with a reality that has no substance, other than the significance assigned to it, has been imagined into existence. Quantum physics seems to suggest that once attention is focused on something with the intention of experiencing it, a highly ordered system of methodical harmonization brings it forth as a unique and personal event. It further proposes that everything that ever was or ever will be is here now in the moment being experienced. But paradoxically, nothing at all exists until it is observed. All of this occurs in an effort to understand the self. This fundamental acknowledgment provides the intellectual basis for every known social structure, relationship, philosophy, and theoretical science that has emerged throughout our history.

All of these evolutionary structures are designed to provide direction, meaning, understanding, and organization for the thoughts entertained, the feelings felt, and the uncertainties universally shared. In essence, all of these efforts simply denote an unquenched thirst for self-realization. They represent different ways of looking at the same thing.

By its very nature, the virtual realm is infinite. It is made up of information, energy, and gaps. These gaps provide the fertile soil of possibility and potential for the eventual emergence of thoughts and experiences. These experiences contribute to memory and desire. Memory begets desire and provides the template for future action resulting in experiences. This substrate offers a prototype for interacting with the primary nature of the virtual realm in a meaningful and personal way that can be refined into a Quantum Lifestyle Dynamic, which we will explore later.

■ Mysteries of the Divine

Soul, ego, mind, intellect, personality, psyche, and countless other words have been fused into instructions for intellectually embracing the notion of virtual vastness. Perhaps the nebulous mystery of the divine has been best encapsulated in the fashionable description of mind-body-spirit. It also forms the foundation for our expanded model. A comprehensive representation of some more familiar attributes can be shaped from this simple, but sophisticated, depiction of the human tri-dimensional nature. These include the basic physical, biochemical, and psycho-emotional-spiritual components of my fundamental model. When fully inflated this classical description exposes the multidimensional character of existence that allows for everything to affect and be affected by everything else. This occurs as a result of the subtle influences generated within the unseen realm by the collective interaction of all people and provides for a look at the veiled reality of the virtual through a different set of eyes.

The human body, in addition to representing the ultimate expression of the other two realms, houses the core components of these realms. Obviously, it provides the structural foundation for movement, stability, perception, interaction, and expression. It also houses the physical brain, spinal cord, nerves, tissues, organs, glands, and functional pathways for the biochemistry. As we will see shortly, the biochemistry provides for a two-way system of communication between and among the realms.

Moving deeper into an exploration of the virtual realm, the first interesting observation is that the brain records information, while the mind experiences it. Subsequently, it would not be unreasonable to assume that the mind, or at least one aspect of it, resides in the brain. This makes the mind a sort of master transformer for the expression of consciousness. Subtle nuances suggesting a less tangible structure with refined functional attributes become visible. It is at this point that the traits assigned to an impression of God begin to materialize. These characteristics encompass attempts to establish a personality profile of the divine.

Supreme, infinite, all knowing, all wise, omniscient, impersonal, and omnipresent are but a few of the descriptive adjectives that have been assigned to the entity associated with the outer reaches of the mind. The other end of the mind is coupled with the brain, which transforms the outer limits of this relationship into practical utilities. These include things such as thoughts, emotions, memories, imaginings, insights, desires, intellect, and creativity, which eventually contribute to personality and ego.

■ The Quest for Self-Realization

While the brain remains autonomous as a distinct entity, it contains one aspect of the mind that is linked to the source of the qualities cataloged above. This occurs through a relationship with a manufactured entity designated as the soul. This suggestion becomes the crossroad of divergent opinions with a common focus relating to the ultimate nature of existence, the purpose of life, and the path to self-realization.

It is at this juncture that many methods, philosophies, beliefs, and religions begin to emerge. These translate as an understanding of divine behavior. They provide a template for interacting with the unseen. Self-realization, then, is not limited to the self of individual egos, but extends to a personal relationship with the divine. It is this relationship that comprises the essence of the tri-dimensional human experience. At the apex of our body-mind-spirit triad resides the intelligence that creates and directs the substance of matter through the mind. In a quest for self-realization, it is less important *how* God is seen, but more so whether God is seen. The prototype that emerges from the words used to describe the character of the unknowable is simply a variation on a theme utilized to establish an account of the virtual.

The effects of the thoughts chosen to create the life being experienced are expressed in the body. So the body is the end result of a process that is a work in progress. In the body resides the ego constructed as an identity based upon beliefs. The biochemistry translates these efforts into feelings and expresses them as emotions stored in the brain as molecules. These subsequently communicate through the soul with the mind in the form of thoughts, desires, and imaginings that link individuals to the formless, timeless, and eternal spirit of the divine.

As spiritual philosopher Ken Wilber so aptly described in one of his essays on witnessing, "Divinity has one ultimate secret, which it will also whisper in your ear if your mind becomes quieter than the fog at sunset." St. Clement clearly stated, "He who knows himself, knows God." But since the divine is indefinable and unknowable, as these expressions disguised as words are deciphered, it is realized that every word has meaning only relative to its opposite. This is merely another way of saying everything is what it isn't. And so, the destination becomes the source. Likewise, the source is the destination. The reality is that they are one in the same. So in being here now, you are already there.

■ The Infinite Nature of the Unseen

Recall that everything affects and is affected by everything else. Also, that thinking makes it so. On a causal level, your best thinking got you where you are today. So the fundamental mechanism for overcoming mental inertia and creating the desired life lies in the quality of thoughts entertained. How can you open your hands to grasp the miracle of your dreams if your arms are full of the past? The secret resides deep in the heart of the final destination—the virtual realm.

According to the classical body-mind-spirit model, everything in the tangible universe is a manifestation of energy and information. Energy and information are the key components of the virtual realm. This means that everything that is thought, done, felt, said, and experienced has its origin in the virtual realm. Exploring this realm presents a challenge, since its organization consists of various elements that are unseen and unseeable except as an effect in the other realms.

These effects originate as energy and are combined with information. Energy vibrates at different frequencies. The higher the vibratory rate, the closer it is to the source of creation. The vibratory rate of an experience determines the nature of the information expressed. Since experience is determined by choices, and choices are dictated by desires, the nature of desires will determine the information ultimately pursued in an effort to define personal reality.

All of the events encountered as part of daily existence originate as part of a dynamic that constitutes the functional reality of the virtual domain. This domain operates beyond the speed of light and far beyond the capability of the senses to identify or process. The conversion of these interactions into physical forms of reality occurs as the potential of the virtual realm is transformed by the body-mind mechanisms into vibratory frequencies that can be perceived through the sensory apparatus.

These end-point receivers, otherwise known as the five senses, represent one aspect of the soul manifest in the mind through the brain as sensory experiences. This quality of being human has been described as the *local self.* It is meant to symbolize the personal and individual interpretation of interaction with the divine. "As above, so below" holds true, with one exception. Expression at this level must be transmitted from a source of pure potential at one end of the mind-spirit relationship, into tangible communication through the mind-body apparatus. In a sense, it becomes a way of divinity communicating with itself, forming a feedback loop for experience, investigation, and evolution.

■ We Are Already Enlightened

If the soul is a manifestation of spirit, and mind is a manifestation of the soul experienced in the body, then enlightenment is articulated in everyday consciousness. By definition, spirit is all encompassing, as being in all things at all times everywhere forever. There is no place it is not, has not been, or will not be. Therefore, the frustration of seeking can be lessened by the knowledge that you are already that which you seek, by virtue of the fact that spirit is also where you are now. To advocate otherwise would mean that you are somewhere spirit is not, and that you must strive to move away from where you are to where it is. But since there is nowhere that it is not, you have only your existing state of awareness in which to experience its expression. For that reason, spirit is always being experienced through the filters of the interpretive apparatus. By its very nature, spirit is constantly experiencing itself through its expression in its experiences. Since spirit is the substance of what it creates, it is contained in what it creates. Because what it creates has the capacity to experience the substance from which it is created, spirit then can experience itself through its own creation. Since spirit constitutes all things, everywhere, all the time, it is also the experience of the moment.

■ Reality as Interpretation

Reality then, as experienced through the *local self,* is an interpretation. At the other end of the spectrum, everyone is united through the mind-spirit aspect of nature to what can be described as a *non-local self.* This *non-local self* can only be described by the characteristics denoted earlier in the discussion of the divine. Infinite and boundless, it exists as all things and nothing. It is the pure spirit from which the universal intelligence operates to unify energy and information into the creative possibilities imagined by the attention of our intentions.

In other words, this "God Force" exists wholly unto itself. This force is self-sufficient and independent. It is available to everyone, according to the extent chosen, to interact with it to co-create the perception of reality experienced. The grain of the mustard seed represents the choice of interaction. It is the door which, if knocked on, will open. It is that which, if asked for, will be received. The caveats established earlier in our discussions could be applied to consciously interact with the creative force that provides the raw materials for the fabrication of individual life experiences. You can start where you are and apply what you know, with the focus of attention on the intention of learning how to consciously co-create the reality of your dreams.

■ An Exercise for Understanding

Perhaps a helpful exercise to network with the virtual might be to look at the type of interactions that have occurred in your life to this point in time. Once understood, the means employed to arrive at the present location can provide the basis for knowing what must be done to reach the destination ultimately desired. To productively observe your present status, it is necessary to examine your personal history and anticipated future. To accurately establish a barometer of conscious interaction with the virtual, in the context of past actions and future aspirations, the concept of time itself must be explored. The nature of this concept can be easily surveyed academically, philosophically, and mathematically. However, the goal of this exploration is to establish a practical application for insight into the human dynamic.

■ Exploring Time

Starting with what is already known, time can be easily understood through a simple dialogue with the senses. The senses operate exclusively in present-time consciousness. For them, through them, and with them, it is impossible to experience any event in the past or in the future. Anything that has already occurred, or anything that has yet to occur, cannot be seen, touched, felt, heard, or tasted. The existing relationship with the virtual consists solely of an ever-changing present that never comes to an end. The only time that we can ever experience is now.

This now is a representation of past decisions, experiences, and encounters. It belongs exclusively to each individual and is solely a personal responsibility. The culmination of these events results in a habitual translation of self-image, personality, appearance, and a feeling of well-being. It also provides the foundation for future action, which will guide and mold who and what you become in the next present moment. This moment subsequently becomes the determining factor in establishing the future present. Within this context, each person is instantly free of victimization, since how one chooses to experience his or her present moments is an entirely personal choice.

Ultimately, the contemplation of who you are now and why you are who you are terminates in a series of contradictions and paradoxes. To a large degree, these revolve around philosophical concepts. These concepts include issues such as free will and fate, life and death, good and evil, absolute and relative. The simple reality is that you are who you are, where you are, experiencing what you are experiencing. Experiences are a result of the interpretation of sensory data assumed in any given moment from the continuum of potential interactions among memories, imaginings and perceptions.

Exploring the practical relevance to our classical body-mind model, an astonishing realization emerges. Despite the intangible roots inherent in the matrix of the virtual, there are some more obvious observations available relative to our constant in-body experiences. Most, if not all, physical experiences of discomfort or pain are directly linked to the virtual through interpretation of the experiences. Despite the fact that discomfort is experienced in the body, the source and the cause lie beyond the material confines of the physical being.

■ Psychosomatic Experiences

This is the basis for the frequently misunderstood discipline of psychosomatic medicine. This discipline is often inappropriately represented as the study of psychological disorders. The behavioral dynamics evaluated within this discipline are more often misconstrued as hypochondria. In fact, hypochondria tends to be more aptly represented by an individual who deliberately, but perhaps unconsciously, creates experiences with behaviors designed to elicit predictable responses that serve an undisclosed need. In contrast, psychosomatic medicine is an invaluable tool for understanding how and why imbalances in the unseen realms can cause an individual to experience physical symptoms that are often misinterpreted to be purely physical disorders.

For example, assume that you have identified an area of your body in which you are experiencing physical discomfort. As the discomfort fails to resolve itself, you become aware that it has progressed into a chronic pain. You then decide to seek evaluation and treatment. A formal assessment results in the diagnosis of a physical disorder. Medication and physical therapy are prescribed. You experience some temporary improvement, but quickly realize that the underlying discomfort continues to persist. You find yourself at the preliminary crossroads of decision-making. Do you accept the diagnosis as part of who you are now in the present moment? Or do you choose to engage in the quest of seeking an alternative explanation for the cause of your discomfort?

In choosing to accept the diagnosis, you agree to accept someone else's opinion concerning the source and nature of a physical discomfort within your own body. Symptoms such as neck pain, back pain, numbness, and tension lend themselves more readily to an understanding of this psychosomatic mechanism. But are you willing to accept a diagnosis of diabetes, cancer, heart disease, or arthritis as a more complicated version of the same dynamic?

In the absence of an acute and obvious trauma, the more common symptoms simply represent areas of chronic misuse. Typically, these are associated with overuse, positional stress, muscle imbalance, or unexpressed emotions. The first three causes can usually be identified and remedied relatively simply. The last one is more difficult and more common.

Most people experience some form of tightness, tension, stiffness, soreness, or pain in some part of their body, which they readily accept and acknowledge. In the absence of overt trauma or debilitating persistence, these symptoms are rarely explored beyond the temporary annoyance of the inconvenience they present. Unless they progress into more problematic obstacles, they are often just accepted and accommodated. More frequently than not, this chronic physical discomfort represents something much more. It is often linked to the ego personality. This entity emerges over a period of years in response to our interaction with the environment, stress, and genetics.

Fundamentally, the manner in which this develops closely parallels the adaptive responses to impulses and emotions. Most frequently, this mechanism involves the response of denial. Denial results from a chronic tendency to avoid responsibility for thoughts, words, actions, and their succeeding circumstances.

In a sense, awareness of tendencies found to be repulsive or determined to be socially unacceptable is suppressed. Since body and mind are not separate in their influence, both are impacted by these decisions. The net result is projected out into the world for others to encounter. Meanwhile, unless these self-constructed demons are confronted, they will continue to remain troublesome in some way, shape, or form, usually as physical discomfort, impairment, or disability.

■ How This All Works

When an impulse or emotion is denied, avoided, or resisted, an expression of a natural response to a situation, experience or encounter is essentially suppressed. In so doing, the foundation for a psychosomatic reflex is assembled, which will ultimately be communicated through the bodily expression of physical discomfort.

Take, for example, the feelings of hostility, resentment, anger, or rage. In choosing how to discharge them, external expressions such as screaming, yelling, physically striking out, or otherwise expressing discontent might be considered. Choosing not to express them may cause them to be confined within the body and restrict the associated muscular behaviors. This involves intentionally preventing a physical demonstration of emotional restlessness by activating voluntary muscle groups to restrict a physical response to an undesirable experience.

This stands in stark contrast to the millions of involuntary reactions to the deliberate, albeit subconscious, efforts to suppress a voluntary response. Herein, lies the mechanism by which imbalances in the form of compensation begin to develop in the other realms. Repeated contact with behavior-producing stimuli causes a pattern of response to become established as a vicious cycle of reaction.

Inevitably, this results in a conflict between muscles trying to express an emotional response and others trying to prevent this expression. The net result is tension in the associated muscle groups. Perpetuated over a period of time, this becomes a habitual conditioned response contributing to chronic congestion in the associated areas. It also results in a blockage directly connected to muscular tension and chronic physical pain.

■ Mind and Body Function Together

Fundamentally, any chronic pain associated with a blockage is caused by voluntarily activating specific muscle groups in an attempt to restrict the expression of some impulse, feeling, or emotion determined to be forbidden, inappropriate, or socially unacceptable. There are some simple and effective ways to manage and remove these blockages that will be discussed shortly. But, for now, simply recognize that the mind and body do not function separately. When an emotion, feeling, or impulse is repeatedly suppressed, a similar effect is produced in the body. Remember the caveat: "For every action, there is a reaction."

Repeatedly suppressing the awareness or expression of a feeling—hostility, for instance— causes a related experience of external oppression to be produced. This may even result in associated feelings of fear, anxiety, or depression. But more to the point, the act of stifling feelings like anger, fear, or hostility will activate muscles in areas linked to the act of holding these experiences in to produce chronic tension. Most commonly, this process involves the muscles of the jaw, throat, neck, shoulders, and upper back. The symptoms produced are frequently those of chronic headaches and neck pain.

Common symptom patterns can also be related to psychosomatic reflexes. This means that chronic non-organic back pain can involve the feeling of being held back. Fighting the urge to strike out can produce shoulder pain. Holding back something that really needs to be said can be displayed as jaw, neck or headache pain. Treating these symptoms usually produces only temporary relief because the source of the tension is rooted in the unseen realm and not the neuromuscular system. Since it is usually not recognized that the symptoms are actually self-created, it is assumed that they are just happening. Subconsciously, the role of a helpless victim being assaulted by forces beyond our control is assumed. The bottom line is that reality, as it is commonly known, is created inside each of us from the raw materials constituting the virtual realm through the perception of the senses. The tools for identifying and resolving these symptoms will be discussed as we assemble our quantum lifestyle.

■ The Role of Genetics

The genetic potential for experience is inherited. Everyone is born with certain unexpressed tendencies that are dependent upon the environment and associated stresses, which contribute to the full revelation of latent aptitudes. On the other hand, these tendencies can be provoked into existence by repeatedly entertained thoughts and routinely spoken words. The choices made in these two arenas impact the genetic tendencies. They also provide the freedom to determine how the results of the interaction will be experienced. Therefore, life is dictated by both destiny and freewill.

Certain genetic traits and characteristics come with the territory of being born into this world as human beings. These genetic tendencies further refine the infinite possibilities available into probabilities. Given the appropriate circumstances, these probabilities can be set into motion and expressed in individual lives. They are a form of generational inheritance received as part of the human birthright. This can play a powerful role in determining an individual's looks, feelings, attractions, cravings, and ultimate evolution.

They are like seeds sown into our particular bloodline, similar to those spawned by any flowering organism. Just like any other seed, they require certain specific conditions to proliferate. In the case of the human organism, these conditions include two broad categories of influence. One is the environment in which we are nurtured and raised. The other is the nature of the stress subjected to during our maturation process.

■ Repetitive Thought Disorders

Environment and stress combine to fertilize the soil of potential Vicious Cycle Disorders. Together, these two elements nurture the offspring comprising the residents of each individual's daily 60,000 thought population. This pattern of conditioned responses can more specifically be referred to as a "Repetitive Thought Disorder." As previously discussed, despite the fact that these thoughts occur in the present, they encompass many memories and hopes. The more there are, and the more frequently they are entertained, the more they dominate personal reality. The interplay of memory and anticipation constantly intersects as part of a larger dynamic to fuel present experiences. But it also provides for an illusory perception of distance. Molded further by the influence of a similar energetic occurring in the lives of everyone else on the planet, a false sense of disorientation and uncertainty regarding our own well-being is experienced. A deep-seated feeling of loneliness begins to emerge.

■ Obstacles to Fulfillment

One of the major obstacles to experiencing a life of fulfillment and contentment is a deep-seated sense of separation. This feeling of separateness occurs almost spontaneously in adolescence as a function of normal development. It is actually an aspect of awareness gone awry. In its early stages, it begins as the recognition of individuality and uniqueness. The distinction between I, me, mine, you, and yours begins to surface as an issue. This realization is fueled by various essentials of the infantile environment. This environment not only includes where one lives, what they have, and what they are exposed to, but who is present in this environment and how they interact with each other and others who live in the immediate surroundings.

In essence, this early "soil" into which everyone is planted consists of everything they are exposed to and taught by those assigned to tend to development and growth. These are the formative years. During this time, rudimentary personality features are cultivated that provide a foundation for the basic operating system of future interactions with society and the universe at large. To a high degree, this is the time when anxiety, which is associated with an awareness of separation, sets the stage for many future adult disorders. The learned behaviors for functioning and coping have their roots in this critical formative period.

It is during this period of time that seemingly well-intentioned manipulation occurs. Control, criticism, flattery, inferiority, anger, resentment, depression, self-doubt, and self-worth fan the flames of the emerging protective device called anxiety. Even at this stage of development, it is possible to lose touch with the creative process, as preoccupation with protecting oneself from the destructive components of the environment becomes a priority. This armoring further perpetuates segregation from the spontaneity of conscious choice and establishes associated beliefs, behaviors, and habits that ultimately interfere with the ability to consciously co-create from a virtual source. It also contributes to the formation of an independent ego.

■ Misunderstanding Separation

The feeling of separateness that distinguishes the ego is simply a matter of misidentifying the self as the body, accomplishments, or possessions. It contributes to a false sense of self-importance that dictates who people think they are. It consumes enormous energy in an effort to constantly improve the physical appearance, forcing more achievement and more acquisitions. All the while, self-comparison to everyone else magnifies the discontent. In so doing, the distance from true potential is exaggerated by feelings of self-doubt and inadequacy. This distracts from the qualities and abilities necessary to establish and maintain a relationship with the source of life and the limitless promise that accompanies it.

In recognizing this, it becomes obvious that we are hiding from ourselves in an identity we have constructed to convince ourselves that we are separate from God. The better defined this individual identity, the further one drifts from knowing his or her true self. The personality, which develops as a result of beliefs about how much separation exists, ultimately emerges as the ego. In effect, the quest for self-awareness establishes an individual as his or her own worst enemy. That is to say, God realizes himself through an individual personality and extinguishes his expression when individual behavior is off-purpose.

■ Losing Sight of Choice

At this point, one begins to lose sight of present-time consciousness and starts to dwell in the past-future phase of their potential. This "choice-less" aspect of the multidimensional constitution provides the entrance fee for the experience of daily existence. Since the best predictor of future behavior is past behavior, a future based upon a distorted memory of the past is falsely assumed. This is a present time recollection of a past-present forming an anticipation of a future-present.

The actual mechanism of this dynamic operates in the current present, shaping the experience upon which opinions are based concerning identity and future outcomes. Common influences mingle to shape a continuum of whole parts, which combine into new wholes. In essence, a part from the past-present is combined with a part of the future-present to form a "partole," or a new whole constructed from parts of a fuzzy past and a projected future. All of this occurs in the present moment of experience. And yet, the whole of that experience is but a part contributing to the whole of potential experiences available to everyone sharing this time and place.

Personality and ego begin to emerge from this process as core operating systems for interacting with the outside world. At this point, separateness from everything and everyone is seemingly confirmed. The false assumption that defensive mechanisms must be employed as a safeguard from being hurt, disappointed, and deprived becomes a priority. An addiction to the supposition of isolation in a world of random events subsequently emerges. Having been taught, told, advised, scolded, and reprimanded by others in the environment who believe this is the way things are, "succumb and cooperate" becomes the motto of an instinctual survival apparatus.

Given the dynamics at work in this stage of one's evolutionary experience, this is not an unreasonable response to the early circumstances into which some people have been thrust. Unfortunately, it is a gross distortion of reality perpetrated by the limited perceptions of the stewards of youth. This distortion is widely disseminated by a society of well-developed ego personalities dependent upon the survival of this belief to maintain the integrity of their own security. This represents the status quo upheld in every aspect of civilization. It is a mutually agreed upon belief system established by the ruling class and nurtured by the organizations, structures, and behaviors adopted for the common good. It is the operating system of the physical world designed to maintain orderliness, stability, compliance, and control.

■ Repressive Nurturing

As part of a well-intended nurturing process, humans are taught how to behave, how to act, what to say, think, do, and believe. Firmly entrenched in this constructed behavior by the age of four or five years old, the more spontaneous, carefree, and creative qualities of our youthful legacy withers from a lack of attentiveness. Soon, it is necessary to become "responsible," but unfortunately, for all the wrong things, in all the wrong ways. In a quest for eternal perfection, it becomes virtually impossible to recognize that struggles and strife are self-constructed and self-imposed—born of an ever-more convincing belief based on separateness, loneliness, and isolation. What is focused on expands, and what is resisted becomes stronger. Suddenly, any "spiritual remnants" are confined to a short period of required visitation performed in a facility associated with a chosen religious preference. During this prescribed phase of penance and reflection, prayers are offered for forgiveness, strength, favor, and relief from the self-created reality of a life to which we fully intend to return shortly after our brief rendezvous with the divine.

Between these fleeting interludes with the "God out there," the status quo is to become immersed in the sensory addiction of an objective material world. This fragmented world is fully constructed from the same essentials available for use as resources in constructing any chosen reality. However, all too often, the choices revolve around an opportunity to recreate defensively along the path of least resistance, in an effort to avoid pain, suffering, torment, terror, and insecurity.

Personal creation is based upon a learned belief in some form of perceived lack, insufficiency, conflict, or fear of death. The lack may consist of inadequate physical amenities, attributes, emotional deficits, or psychological insecurities. The hidden hope is for comfort, peace, pleasure, and security. And yet, daily behaviors are enacted that support and perpetuate the probability of experiencing just the opposite. Conversely, it is these adopted behaviors that provide the salve of relief and comfort in the imagined world of random discontent.

■ Sensory Satisfaction

Sensory addictions are meager compromises adopted as transitory substitutes for long-forgotten feelings that we are unable to re-establish or maintain. Because the senses are tangible, available, and relatively easy to pacify in the short term, something is found that feels good and is often repeated, or new sources of stimulation to appease masked cravings are endlessly sought out. But these vain, futile efforts to achieve a perpetual state of well-being are fleeting attempts to satisfy an appetite that resides in a different realm. Therefore, there is no *thing* that will ever provide for the sense of well-being we are striving for. However, there is something that will.

■ Ever-Present Awareness

Eons of sages from every spiritual discipline have suggested that there is something in everyone that is always conscious. It is this ever-present awareness that is the creative force from which we all have emerged. It is the all-pervasive intelligence that sustains and nurtures the very existence we experience. It is this spirit from which all of us come and to which all of us return that stands waiting to receive and respond to the most heartfelt

requests. It is this underlying current of endless consciousness that maintains the order in the universe and awaits an invitation to rejoin the individual experience of life as a co-conspirator in the fulfillment of deep desires
and longings. One has only to identify this relationship lost through lack of
attention to realize that the kingdom of heaven is truly within each of us.

As individual awareness is expressed, we realize that a reunion with the
part of personal identity that is eternal, timeless, and constant is what is
being sought. That enduring personality resides in the virtual realm. The
virtual realm resides in the kingdom of heaven. The virtual realm is the
kingdom of heaven. The link through the body and the mind to the virtual
allows an opportunity to realize and express our divine nature. This is
accomplished through pathways designed for access by the same means
employed to create the reality currently being experienced. The only difference is that conscious participation produces a much more desirable
result.

■ Doorway to the Divine

Access is directly granted by attention and intention. Remember, what is
given attention expands. So focusing attention creates an intention. Eventually, the ability to intentionally and spontaneously manifest what is
desired into being can be willfully developed. Tracing the source of attention, it is realized that the fundamental goal is to experience pleasure and
avoid pain. This is accomplished through choices. Everyone is already
functioning as a full-time creator of his or her own experiences, so learning
to do it effectively and consistently in as specific a way as possible is effort
well spent.

We'll talk in more detail about this core concept in the chapter on Quantum Lifestyle Dynamics. There, we will construct a personal program for
improving the experience of life. For now, simply recognize that the quality of a relationship with the spiritual essence is inextricably bound to the
physical reality of our daily experience. Also note that the beliefs held true
concerning the nature of the divine dictate the quality of that relationship.

■ All Means All

So, too, will this awareness soften a relationship with the divine nature of the multidimensional existence we experience. Regardless of personal beliefs about the nature of God, the qualities, characteristics, and attributes associated with this name are universally accepted as part of its personality. To acknowledge a deity that is infinite, all-knowing, omnipresent, all-powerful, eternal, and everlasting is to affirm that those same qualities permeate one's own innate character. Everyone is mysteriously linked through the soulful aspect of the mind to divinity at all times. However unattainable these traits may seem, they are an inherent aspect of the process of transformation. This transformation is accelerated when priorities are reconfigured to include the spiritual.

The virtual realm is construed to be "out there," or assigned to "the hereafter." However, for the virtual to exist as an entity with the assigned qualities and characteristics, a simple shift in perception can unmask its unavoidable presence. It is easily recognizable as a natural part of evolution operating beyond gene pools and belief systems to create, sustain, and propagate all of creation. Once achieved, this perceptual shift prescribes the personal responsibility of choice as a means for consciously interacting with the process of creation.

The nature and frequency of these choices blend to produce familiar actions and reactions that ultimately coalesce into familiar patterns of behavior and conviction. Further choices molded by an intention to remain flexible will provide the opportunity for unique experiences of the ever-changing collective exposure to external influences. These choices will enhance our ability to look at things differently, ensuring that the things looked at will change. Ultimately, this approach will diminish the impact of unexpected encounters to assure that the importance is placed upon an ability to consciously choose a response, rather than allowing the event encountered to dictate an outcome.

And so, each person paints from the palate of possibilities the portrait of their own lives. One may draw from the infinite influences available in the virtual realm to construct a unique masterpiece constructed upon the genetic framework of their DNA and shaped by the collective forces of environment and choices. This, then, is the face of the virtual.

To this point, an outline has been constructed for appreciating who we are, how we function, and why we do what we do. Within this context, it is relatively easy to examine many other issues that have plagued mankind unceasingly. The dynamics of many contemporary interactions can be understood, if not explained away, when superimposed upon the tri-dimensional model of being human. Lucid explanations can now be proposed for the larger questions of where did we come from, what happens when we die, why does evil exist, and why do bad things happen to good people? However, they remain fodder for philosophical discourse, unless a personal experience of the underlying dynamics can be cultivated and applied to improve individual lives.

In other words, it's good and helpful to engage the matters of good and evil, the nature of God, and relationships with the divine. It's certainly interesting to understand the miraculous energetic of the human body and the inner workings of the mind. It's even useful to construct a model of practical spirituality as a guide through the gauntlet of daily life. But, in the final analysis, one must ask if this is just fascinating reading material, or if it can be used by the average human being to establish control over individual circumstances in creating a gratifying personal experience?

■ A Model for Change

The model upon which the foundation for change is based is rooted in the original age-old design of the human organism. It is interesting to marvel at the saga of a fully formed human organism. On a microscopic level, this process metaphorically mimics the life experience of a human being.

Genetically, the human life form emerges from a single cell, which replicates only fifty times before dividing into 250 different species. Each performs millions of independently related functions per second.

What happens next is no less intriguing, as each cell replies to outside environmental influences. This reaction produces responses that contribute to the creation of a functional biochemical personality. This personality includes an involuntarily learned behavior that results in experiences that produce desires. These desires form intentions and create attention, predisposing us to a recurring series of events.

■ The Spectrum of Being

Within the constructs of the proposed prototype, human potential can be understood and appreciated. As spirit emerges from timelessness through the thick of virtual possibilities, it expresses itself as the soul of mankind. This soul has one foot always securely rooted in the virtual. It communicates through the mind to the brain, which translates throughout the biochemistry portrayed in physical form as the human body. This is the spectrum of being and consciousness. In this model of reality, the universal consciousness inhabits its own creation and experiences existence through what it creates. So, too, it seeks an awareness of itself in that which it creates.

Inherent in the nature of that which is sought, is a virtual variable to the quest at hand. This variable is a paradox of sorts. A subtle and disturbing insight emerges as the larger premise of this sojourn toward the divine is pondered. God, by definition, is ever-present, in all things, everywhere, at all times. Therefore, there is nowhere, at anytime, that God is not. Given this philosophical quandary, it is a short intellectual leap to the conclusion that a search may be futile. Given the definition above, everyone already is and has everything that could ever be desired, since we too, are one of the places where God always exists. Therefore, what is being sought after is something already established and possessed. But how is this possible?

By definition, this creative intelligence exists beyond time and space. It always existed, everywhere, in everyone, and will continue to do so for eternity. In that context, if all things are part of this endless awareness, there are no longer things apart from it. Taking this a step further, everyone would necessarily originate from a common source expressing different qualities and characteristics through unique personalities. In this sense, there is really no difference between any of us; together we form one solitary organism.

Therefore, what affects one of us, affects all of us. Separation exists only in the illusion of individual human forms. The quest for the "one taste", described by noted author and philosopher Ken Wilber, is inhibited only by the development of the ego personality, which convinces us that because of our unique gifts, talents, trials, tribulations, and experience, we are separate from each other and estranged from our source. But the reality is that we actually only share different flavors of the same taste. Our unique and individual contributions to the collective influence of our multidimensional existence dictates, determines, and ensures a privileged personal experience.

■ Applying Principles of Change

To fully appreciate the magic available in any proposed process, one must apply acceptable principles to their own lives. Unless this information can be applied and related to individual lives in a way that allows for an experience of the miracle of creation, this whole exercise will amount to little more than another brief moment of inspiration that temporarily quenches a passionate longing for purpose, meaning, and contentment.

Change is inevitable. But the simple question remains: Will you continue to be a victim of change, or will you choose to experience the changes you create for yourself? It is at this junction that a new decision must be made. Since change is inevitable and life goes on, how will you choose to go on with your life? From within the tri-dimensional experience of a multidimensional existence, it is likely for one to emerge from the virtual recognizing that who is not yet enlightened pales in comparison to those who are not yet aware that they are. Realizing that who one chooses to be influences the choices of others, and that others contributing to the collective whole provide everyone with the same opportunity, it is quickly recognized that the only thing anyone can do for anyone else is to work on themselves.

And so, departing from the virtual forever changed, encouraged, motivated, and confident, the final frontier back to personal reality is left to be traversed. All that remains is to synthesize a new understanding into a functional awareness that will constitute the operating system of a Quantum Lifestyle Dynamic. But first we must take a look at how our choices contribute to the experience of recurring symptoms known as VCD.

Ready for a Change?

■ Now is the time to begin, because there is no time but now.

■ When you change the way you look at things, the things you look at change.

■ As you think, so will be your experience.

■ What you experience is not nearly as important as how you experience it.

■ The only thing you can do for anyone else is work on yourself.

■ CHAPTER FOUR ■
Anatomy of a Realm

"We are at the very beginning of time for the human race. It is not unreasonable that we grapple with problems. But there are tens of thousands of years in the future. Our responsibility is to do what we can, learn what we can, improve the solutions, and pass them on."

—RICHARD FEYNMAN, U.S. EDUCATOR AND PHYSICIST (1918–1988)

The word *realm* can simply mean an area. It can also be used to describe a domain, a kingdom, a monarchy, an empire, or a territory. When I talk about realms, I am referring to distinct attributes associated with the various aspects of human experience. As I indicated in the introduction to this book, human experience is multidimensional. This means that there are a lot of different aspects and components that interact to produce an overall encounter with life.

There are numerous subcategories to each realm and numerous words used to describe the various aspects of existence. I have chosen to use a simplified and generic model. This model has not been adopted to the exclusion of others, nor is it designed to alienate, criticize, condemn, or ostracize any individual belief or perspective. To the contrary, it is an attempt to express a unified perspective that transcends any words that might be used to describe reality as I have observed and experienced it.

■ Reality of the Realms

Each realm has certain characteristics that make it unique. Yet, all of the realms intersect to produce a totally distinctive experience known as life. When examining a realm, its nature will be analyzed. This includes the way that it looks, functions, and interacts with the other realms. In doing so, a world of endless possibilities inevitably materializes. This includes all the things that can go wrong within the realm, or that can affect its behavior.

I have arbitrarily assigned names to the realms in an effort to reference their sphere of influence aside from the manner in which they interact with the others. For instance, while the physical realm possesses distinct qualities, it also affects, and is affected by, the other two realms. In addition, the cumulative dynamic of each person is affected by contact with other people experiencing their multidimensional lives. But it doesn't end there. The collective interaction of all of the elements in all of the realms experienced by all individuals produces a communal consciousness from which emerges an influential pattern of behavior and probability.

This pattern of behavior is observed in the unspoken agreements entered into while the daily activities of any given society are conducted. It is reflected in the laws enacted to supervise the collective code of demeanor. It is the basis for all of the customs and ways of life in any given culture or civilization. This pattern of probability suggests the likelihood that a given phenomenon will occur. It dictates the nature of the status quo. In other words, if this is the way things have always been done, it is most likely that they will continue to be done that way. This dynamic will be explored in detail throughout the remainder of the book. For the moment, a closer look at the anatomy of each realm is essential.

■ The Physical Realm

The physical realm is the easiest realm to relate to since we wake up in it everyday and function all day long with it as a constant companion. We wash it, primp it, exercise it, rest it, and take it places that it will enjoy.

Sometimes we derive pleasure from engaging it in things that are ultimately harmful for it, such as eating too many sweets, staying up too late, or lying in the sun on the beach all day. Nonetheless, the body is designed as a vehicle to transport us from birth to death and everywhere in between. However, it is so much more than just a vehicle. With all of its finely tuned components and unexpressed potential, it is capable of providing us with a medium for self-awareness and transcendence.

When considered as an individual entity, the human body first appears as a compilation of cells, tissues, organs, glands, and systems. In light of the time-honored assumptions of conventional medical dogma, all of these components can be statistically categorized. The progression and outcome of the physical body can be accurately predicted; that is to say, everyone is going to grow old and die. Despite this conventional cornerstone of "scientific medicine," it is really about the only thing that is reasonably predictable. Upon closer inspection, we see gross contradictions to this traditional wisdom. Perhaps aging and death are inevitable, but the quality of life experienced in the interim is not nearly as predictable as once thought.

■ Brain Science

Take, for example, the conviction of orthodox subscribers to the model of brain degeneration. Deterioration of brain cells is not only accepted, it is said to be inevitable and predictable. According to this paradigm, aging is associated with smaller, lighter brains, lacking the necessary physical circuitry to maintain functional integrity. However, contemporary research provides common examples of individuals who were unaware that this was supposed to take place. Further scrutiny reveals a dynamic that implies a dissimilar probability. The "new reality" suggests that as long as individuals subject themselves to sufficient external stimulation, they can remain as intelligent and as mentally active while aging as they were at any point in their lives.

Remember, even though everything that ever existed, or ever will exist, exists right now, nothing at all exists until it is observed. Innovative technology provides the tools for observing the activity of structures in the human body that were previously inconceivable; and yet, once observed, it's hard to believe that the earlier data were not previously available.

■ Mind over Matter

Humbled by the complex simplicity with which the human organism thrives and perpetuates itself, the true inference of mind over matter can be conceded. Despite the theoretical controversy surrounding the practical presumption of what controls what, in the final analysis, the universe is constructed of energy and information. While matter and energy are undeniably interchangeable, matter is created from energy, and the movement of energy governs the function of matter. One needs to look no further than the brain itself to see a demonstration of this in action.

■ Unreal Realities

The impressions you form during this process of living and growing are based upon the assumption that you perceive the world as it actually exists. However, the underlying reality may be constructed upon an entirely different set of facts. Once known, they may suggest an alternative interpretation.

Direct perception of the physical world is mediated through your senses. Scientific investigation suggests that there is a delay of about one fifth of a second between any event in the physical world and your experience of it. Relying exclusively on the sensory images that emerge as a result of contact with an event can lead to an inhibited experience of life. Remember that this is a physical encounter with a material world that is linear in nature and subject to the rules of cause and effect. This means that for every action, there's an equal and opposite reaction that is predictable. If you throw a stone, the height and distance it will travel is predicated upon certain related factors, such as the amount of force used to launch it. It is within this predictable realm that the trajectory of billiard balls and space shuttles can be planned. Similarly, weather forecasts, motor vehicle damage, and interest on invested money can be calculated. The ultimate goal of all scientific investigation is to pierce this veil of predictability in an attempt to isolate the laws and principles that govern their consistency. Thus, you are allowed an opportunity to directly interact with the fundamentals of a given experience to affect the outcome.

On a practical level, when something as unpretentious as a nerve cell is observed, it is easy to draw parallels between its appearance and that of a jellyfish. The countless thin arms radiating from its globular body project out into its surroundings, awaiting contact. Similar to contact with the tentacles of a jellyfish, human nerve cells propel messages to other similar structures in their environment. However, unlike the jellyfish, more than one message is communicated. Imagine this vast network of nerve cells as the telecommunications system of the body. It conveys information to other cells in remote parts of the body and receives critical details about function from other like organisms.

It is classically taught that these nerve cells, called neurons, decline rapidly with age. It is also taught that brain cell death is permanent and that these neurons are incapable of regenerating. It is believed that the rate and number of decline are associated with degenerative diseases of aging, such as senility. In fact, this is merely a corresponding observation. The reality is that, even though these neurons do behave as described in the literature, a related fact is not taken into account. The jellyfish projections, called dendrites, are capable of reproducing and proliferating to compensate for loss of function.

Moreover, the functional integrity of the nervous system is dictated by use, not age. Use it or lose it has never been more appropriately represented than in this example. A related indicator suggests that the structure and function of the nervous system is governed by the availability of raw materials. These raw materials exist in the form of vital nutrients that are indispensable to the basic operation of every task each cell must perform to maintain optimal performance. Assessing the raw materials available for the body to perform all of its necessary functions on a daily basis appears to be a central aspect of any fundamental system review. Since nutrients come from food intake, it is no coincidence that more than 70 percent of all degenerative diseases are linked to diet.

■ Supply and Demand

Think of it like this: If the human body must perform 1,000 functions everyday, but is consistently supplied with only enough raw material to perform 500, then 500 things a day are not going to get done. The body, in its innate wisdom, allocates the available resources to fuel those functions most essential to sustaining life. All other functions become optional and expendable. So to the extent that raw materials are available, the body will cooperate and compensate to accomplish what it can. Everything else is either sacrificed or compromised. It is this process that forms the basis for a biochemical imbalance leading to one form of Vicious Cycle Disorder. It really boils down to supply and demand.

For some reason, the simplicity of this concept has eluded mainstream approaches to restoring and maintaining optimal function of the body. Consider for a moment the 1912 Nobel-Prize-winning work of Alexis Carrel, who kept a chicken heart alive for several decades. He is considered to be the Jules Verne of cardiovascular surgery. His experiment suggested that one of the secrets of life is to feed and nourish cells and allow them to flush their waste and toxins. His work inferred that if you can provide the appropriate nutrition for a cell and remove the waste material, it would never die. In other words, deliver nutrients and eliminate waste and the cells of the body are potentially immortal. This certainly leaves room for considering an overhaul of actuarial tables. His experiment did not end because the chicken heart died. It ended because his point was made and his experiment was terminated. Yet, there has been no practical application of this radical finding in mainstream medicine.

One related concept that warrants additional consideration is that of surface tension. If the surface tension of the fluid in which the nutrients are being transported is too high, the nutrients can't get into the cell and the cellular waste can't get out. Eventually the cells dehydrate and die in a pool of toxic debris. This concept will be revisited when the realm of human biochemistry is explored. At this point, however, the anatomy of the physical realm will establish a starting point for more exotic excursions.

■ Human Anatomy 101

The human body is estimated to contain 50 trillion cells. They look relatively unimpressive, even under a microscope. The anatomy of each of the different cells that comprise the body fills volumes of texts. In reality, although fascinating to study, anatomy remains little more than a container for the magic that happens inside each of the little bags of fluid. Some fundamental facts about physical structure are worthy of note in developing a basic appreciation and understanding for the design and function of the human organism.

The human body is a well-ordered mechanism designed to provide for a means of expression and experience. The systems of the body are well integrated structurally. The skeletal system provides attachments for soft tissues that allow for structural stability and movement. The cranial cavity houses and protects the central processing unit of the spinal cord. The spinal column gives shelter to the spinal cord and provides a conduit for distribution of the spinal nerves, blood vessels, and lymphatic vessels that dwell within. Even the individual cells themselves protectively house vital organisms that are crucial to procreation.

The nerves communicate impulses of information to and from the brain. They provide a means of interaction and control over every minute function in the cells, tissues, organs, and glands. They convey and synchronize data to and from every aspect of our daily physical encounters. They provide a structure for the transport of information between the inside and outside worlds. Despite nerves' obvious influence, their importance is diluted in a medical bias that characterizes the body as primarily material.

■ The Miracle of Renewal

On the other hand, moving beyond the superficial physical form of the body, there is much about which to be amazed. The body is constantly renewing itself. The skin is renewed every month. Every four days a new stomach lining is manufactured. The cells that make up the surface cells of the body renew every five minutes. With the rate of renewal of cells in the liver, a new liver is theoretically produced every six weeks. The bony skeleton regenerates every three months. Ninety-eight percent of the atoms throughout the entire body are completely different than a year ago.

Through the wondrous processes that deliver nutrients and remove waste, the body is constantly under renovation. The rate of exchange varies from system to system. The mechanisms for repair and rejuvenation differ. Nonetheless, this process continues day after day, from birth to death, to create a new you in every moment.

The body, in and of itself, is a true paradox. It is durable, solid and stable. Yet, it remains changeable and fluid, new in every moment. Thus, the physical material aspect of the body is intimately connected to elements of the other realms. This association is not limited by material or biochemical attributes. Nor is it a one-way street. The body exists in a dynamic collaboration of exchange, negotiating input and providing stimulation for the distribution of vital resources to and from its counterparts.

■ Linking the Realms

Aside from its structural anatomy, the human body functions as a medium for interaction with the other realms. The specialized functions of the sensory organs bridge the related biochemical and virtual realms. Peering beneath the veil of what appears to be obvious, a world of information, energy, and vibration is discovered. The anatomy of this unseen world is not dissimilar to that of the structural anatomy of the physical body, but it is one rarely looked at, and one more rarely seen. Complete new realities exist at every level of observation. In fact, no matter where or how this virtual universe is observed, it is filled with things to see as information, and energy abound in infinite capacities.

If we look exclusively at the physical structure of the human body, we see shape, form, beauty, function, and every conceivable expression of emotion, passion, and thought. If we examine the inner workings of the human vehicle, we encounter a world of cells, molecules, atoms, hormones, nutrients, and waste products, as well as structures designed for communication, repair, reproduction, and transportation. Looking deeper, we can observe the effects of the virtual interactions taking place in every moment, in response to every exchange from the physical to the biochemical, emotional, psychological, and beyond.

Looking intently at the physical universe of the human body, a tangible model to dissect and interpret is exposed. Its composition can be observed, and diverse functions can be assigned to isolated systems. However, how it actually works is indescribable. What is seen can be described, but why it is seen cannot. Because of the dynamic inter-relationships of the realms, any attempt to interpret the interactions observed in the body merely becomes yet another graphic insight. What we see is a reflection of the activities produced by the constant exchange of information among the realms. The more the physical realm is observed, the more it resembles the other realms. When examining a cell, its likeness to the organizational structure of the human body becomes more apparent. In fact, all cells, with the exception of red blood cells, contain a nuclear cranial cavity that houses the DNA brain of cellular procreation.

Ultimately, all of the information managed by the body must be processed in the physical brain. But which brain is processing what? Is the physical brain processing data from all of the realms, or is the virtual brain producing responses to stimulation from each realm? Where does the information come from that gets processed? How does it get interpreted and communicated? These questions represent the foundation of the mind-body movement. They also represent the biggest challenge in physical medicine, as the vigorous newness of the body changes in every moment. It is in this very newness that the true potential of future medicine resides. This potential remains to be expressed as we contemplate how it is possible to interact in the moment with something that changes so quickly while we appear to be standing still. All that can be achieved in this setting is to consciously observe. And observe we do.

■ Hidden Intelligence

Beyond the structural confines of gross human anatomy, processes can be observed. These processes have always existed. They advance into awareness as they are observed. Therefore, it is safe to assume that the physical body mirrors an intelligence that created and maintains it in response to our input and exposure. And while the intelligence that inhabits the human body is the same intelligence that created it, this intelligence does not reside exclusively in the body. Consequently, any effort to explore and examine the source of intelligent life renders little more than an opportunity to observe the effects of this intelligence.

The anatomical pathways of human biochemistry demonstrate the means by which events occur, but do not suggest the manner in which they originate. Certainly the responses to stimuli can be observed. However, that which is stimulating remains somewhere between the observed stimulus and the response. A thought, an emotion, a desire, or an impression can be experienced. But little more than a reaction to these intangible events can be observed. To speculate in this area, it is necessary to move, not only beyond medicine, but also beyond science.

CHAPTER FIVE

The River of Life

"Rivers flow from east and west to merge with the one sea, forgetting that they were ever separate rivers. So, it is here that our separateness begins to soften."

—Unknown

■ Crossing the Biochemical Bridge

Moving from the material realm toward the virtual involves crossing the bridge of biochemistry. In crossing, it is recognized that this waterway is a channel of transformation and transportation for the other realms. Matter becomes energy and vice versa. Everything that has been observed up to this point is not everything that can be observed.

■ Similarity of the Realms

Progressing from the physical to the biochemical realm, similarities become evident. The same caveats apply to observations in this realm. The biochemical realm is an ever-changing entity unto itself. It is this unique quality that allows it to be what it isn't. Similarly, it only exists as such when looked at through the eyes of perception. This perception grants occasion to view the residents of this realm as functional counterparts to those of the physical realm. In other words, an assessment of this realm must be considered as a possible source of imbalance potentially contributing to the symptoms being evaluated before a decision to treat is implemented. In essence, the biochemical and physical realms are no different. But by nature, they are a world apart. The cells that comprise the liquid realm of biochemistry are material and real. Technology gives us a glimpse into this world. It allows for the observation of a population motivated by an inexpressible consciousness that conforms to the laws of cause and effect.

Peering deeper into the colonies of cells populating the biochemical realm, things once again look different. The refined mechanisms composing the structure and function of these tiny transformers provide for a close proximity to the virtual realm. Moving beyond the gross structure of the cell itself, the molecules, atoms, and subatomic particles that provide the final link to the virtual realm can be observed once they are considered for possible involvement.

When dealing at this level of awareness, information and energy rule. It is here that an understanding of the true nature of being begins to emerge. Equipped with the caveats and a unique perspective, an assessment of the biochemical realm can unfold by way of additional examples. These will serve as aids in deciphering the hidden secrets of this waterway, while assisting in experiencing the origin of creation's destiny.

The dynamics presiding over the physical realm are self-evident and ever-present in the realm of biochemistry. But they are also much less apparent. The society of this biological kingdom is presided over by energy and information. To appreciate the chain of command in this realm, it is important to recognize the collaborative nature of this environment.

The internal environment of the body is a wet and wild ecosystem full of impeccably ordered frenzy. Millions, if not billions, of interactions occur every second. From the time this world was first considered by researchers, it was believed to be a randomized slush pond that contained the debris from its activity and exposure. The earth and its populace were similarly imagined as being governed by an unseen intelligence. It was believed that these global inhabitants had been programmed by this intelligence from the beginning of time. It was further assumed that the activity of this intelligence was coordinated by the brain and central nervous system of its earthly host.

Time and technology created a window into this world, allowing for observation of its rhythmic exchanges. Fully understanding the significance of these interactions is a work in progress. Not unlike human anatomy, biological fluids eventually demonstrated a similar structural hierarchy. Ultimately, the composition of this ecosystem displayed some fairly predictable characteristics. Generically, it is assumed that molecules and cells comprised the general population of this environment. With the advent of the various specialties in biomolecular medicine, additional structures, organisms, and functions have been identified.

Accordingly, if the external structure of the human body represents material reality, the internal environment represents functional reality. But once again, everything is what it isn't! Physical existence has physiology or function that is discernible. So, too, physiology has structure inherent in its composition. However, regardless of the name assigned to this internal maze of motion, it remains an integral part of the human experience.

■ Inner Workings of the Matrix

This interior planet of liquid commotion has been referred to as the biological terrain and the internal milieu. I have named this setting the *biological matrix* and will refer to it as such throughout the remainder of this discussion. I have also assigned the depiction of matrix transformation to the processes occurring here.

The gross anatomy of the biological systems consists of vessels, organisms, cells, molecules and subatomic particles. Superficially this environment functions as a medium where chemical reactions occur. So, too, nutrients and waste products are transported and stored here. More simplistically, the function of this system is comparable to the fundamental nature of the chicken heart experiment. Optimal balance is maintained when the proper ratio of nutrients in and waste products out is preserved. But as with all things, when you look at them differently, they look different. And there's much more here than meets the eye.

■ Surface Tension

Earlier, I briefly mentioned a concept referred to as surface tension. In fact, this is far more than a concept. It is a phenomenon that serves as an invisible, but observable, barrier between the external membrane of all the cells in the body and the outside world. It is the ultimate buffer between what gets into the cells and what gets out. Now, there are numerous other mechanisms that participate in the process of assimilation and excretion, but surface tension rules in determining how efficiently these mechanisms perform their functions at any given time.

■ The Bottom Line

Surface tension is an observable fact that is often dealt with in daily life without realizing it. The cohesive forces between liquid molecules are responsible for this phenomenon. The molecules at the surface unite to form a surface film, which makes it more difficult to move an object through the surface than to move it when it is completely submersed.

Surface tension is typically measured in dynes/cm, the force in dynes required to break a film of 1 cm in length. Water at 20°C has a surface tension of 72.8 dynes/cm. This simple fact has both clinical and practical applications. For instance, in the real world, the major reason for using hot water for washing is that its surface tension is lower and it is a better wetting agent. But if a detergent lowers the surface tension, the heating may be unnecessary. There are many other examples that demonstrate the effects of surface tension in day-to-day reality, but fascinating as they are, there is one extremely important aspect to this concept that pertains to our personal biochemistry.

The surface tension of ordinary tap water is approximately 73 dynes/cm. The surface tension of extra cellular body fluids is much lower at approximately 40 dynes/cm. This low surface tension is critical to healthy cellular function, absorption of nutrients, and the removal of toxins.

For the body to access the contents of the ingested fluids and eliminate cellular waste efficiently, the surface tension of that fluid must be reduced to as close to the surface tension of the bodily fluids as possible. For this to occur, one of two things must take place. One is that some agent must be added prior to ingestion to reduce the surface tension of the fluid. The other is that the body must expend energy to reduce the surface tension of the fluid after it has been ingested. If the body is already functioning with limited resources, the energy expended on this process will be restricted, and the ability to absorb and eliminate waste will be compromised.

Therefore, three things must be considered to ensure the efficient function of this mechanism. First, the integrity of the basic operating capacity of the body must be evaluated and enhanced. Secondly, it is important to use a source of drinking water with a surface tension as close as possible to the surface tension of bodily fluids. Finally, the existing water source can be supplemented with an additive capable of reducing the surface tension.

■ More Than a Medium

Upon further inspection, our biological system is utilized for far more than just a medium, a transport system, or a storage facility. It is a second nervous system, functioning as a transformer for the transmutation of energy into information. It is a channel of communication between the physical and virtual realms. But before going into that, some further definitions are in order to accurately map out the terrain of this soggy kingdom. Since the two major inhabitants of this biochemical region are cells and molecules, a descriptive exploration of each is in order. Cells are essentially little bags filled with chemicals and water. Different cells look differently under a microscope and perform different functions.

Now all of these little fluid filled bags, with the exception of red blood cells, contain a fundamental structure called a nucleus. The nucleus houses and protects our DNA. There are many other structures within the cell that perform highly specialized functions incidental to this discussion. Even so, each cell performs millions of activities while contributing to the multitude of functions required by the tissue, organ, or gland in which it resides. The infinite number of coordinated activities occurring in the human body is orchestrated by an invisible intelligence residing in the virtual realm. However, its presence is only observed by means of its activity. The resident neighbor of the cell is the molecule.

A molecule is the tiniest possible piece of a substance that can still be identified as that substance. These molecules are composed of smaller units. These units, called atoms, are the smallest units of matter. Atoms are substances such as hydrogen, nitrogen and carbon. These atoms are bound together in a configuration specific to a substance. Chemical formulas, equations, and diagrams all represent the authenticity of these configurations. These molecules are attracted to each other by an invisible intelligence to form identifiable substances and structures. In fact, cells are made of molecules. These molecules are the part of the mechanism of communication that qualifies this biological organism as the second nervous system.

The bag-like exterior of the cell is also known as the cell membrane. This membrane is saturated with tiny molecules called receptors. These receptors are the equivalent of the physical body's senses in the cellular environment. They pick up chemical messages sent from everywhere in the body and communicate the transmission into the internal environment of the cell for processing and response. A chain reaction of biochemical events then occurs, causing changes in the immediate environment. These events translate into thought, activity and feelings, as a result of the transformations that take place within the biological matrix.

■ Mysteries of the Matrix Revealed

Only recently has this matrix been acknowledged for its dramatic impact on who we are or how we perform as a whole person. Previously, the biological matrix was regarded as a reservoir of inactivity, serving merely as a switching post for the more complicated proceedings of the organs and glands. Long before the biological matrix was identified as an organism of significance, the brain and the central nervous system were thought of as a mere electrical telegraph system. The chemical brain was all but nonexistent until things were looked at in a different way. In all fairness to the researchers of that time, the tools for observing these phenomena were yet to be developed.

Since when all you have is a hammer, everything looks like a nail, the nervous system was viewed as an elaborate maze of exotic wiring. After all, a typical neuron (nerve cell) looks like a cross between a tadpole and a porcupine. Nerves provide for the hierarchy of communication in the human body, but long before nervous systems and brains even existed, chemical substances supplied the basis for communication inside cells. All the same, it was well accepted during this period of "telegraph system consciousness" that tiny chemicals jumped from cell to cell, providing "on" and "off" instructions throughout the nervous system.

The foundation for much of the current understanding of the brain, the nervous system, chemicals of communication, and the equilibrium of internal biochemical processes was laid in the late nineteenth and early twentieth centuries. Each passing decade brought the reality of these environments into clearer focus and brought the divergent specialties ever so much closer together. Eventually, researchers could no longer ignore the fact that for every question, there is an answer, for every problem, a solution, and for every chemical, a receptor. The 1970s and 1980s supplied the impetus to move beyond this simplistic understanding of brain and nervous system function.

Current thinking suggests that the physical brain has both electrical and chemical features. These features allow for the transmission of information via electrical discharges. This occurs at the junction between two nerve cells and via substances called neuropeptides that bind to specific receptors on cells throughout the entire body.

Generations of researchers have contributed to these discoveries. However, I would be remiss if I did not acknowledge the work of one very special neuroscientist who brought it all together in its current form. Candace Pert, Ph.D. discovered a structure called the opiate receptor in 1972. This discovery provided the quantum leap necessary for today's current understanding of the brain and nervous system. In her book, *Molecules of Emotion: The Science Behind Mind-Body Medicine*, she established the biomolecular basis for emotions. This work embodies the essence of the journey beyond medicine. It is a well-established fact that the body is a sophisticated pharmacy, capable of manufacturing chemicals yet to be identified. It's when these chemicals get congested in the matrix, don't get produced in sufficient quantities, or get used up or otherwise impaired, that we experience emotional upset.

▪ The Illusion of Confusion

On the other hand, the body is able to self-regulate experiences of pain through the matrix by overriding the pain signals. Any circumstance that distracts or diverts our attention is a good example of how this is accomplished. Remember, attention produces intention, which produces experience. So, too, by this very mechanism, the body responds to attention through the matrix. In doing so, it allows for the experience of desirable outcomes to occur despite the presence of a pain-producing experience. Take attention away from the pain, and the pleasure of not feeling pain is experienced.

Common examples might be those in which an individual is faced with an emergency situation to which they must respond to preserve a life. More common examples might be the diversion of attention away from a recent cut or a sore back while engaged in an activity of concentrated interest. The chemicals that mediate this dialog in the matrix are the equivalent of verbal dialogue. They are silent, but they speak nonetheless. It is the same process performed without conscious participation. Intelligence transformed into its material counterpart through biochemistry brings us one step closer to consciously manifesting our intent in the day-to-day experience of life.

■ All in Your Head

Before long, all of the "all in your head" experiences will be formally associated with their biochemical counterparts. The next leap will take us into the virtual realm, where participation in the conscious creation of reality is possible. This mechanism is alive and well, however its delicate intricacies go unnoticed. As the body mirrors its mental activities, numerous changes are produced in response to the thoughts one chooses. The conscious creation of personal reality through the diligent exercise of the virtual realm is now more than just wishful thinking.

Well-known is the fact that the body and the mind are not separate. Numerous research projects suggest evidence to support this proposition. Since the same chemical substances and receptors exist throughout the entire colony of cells, every aspect of physical being is capable of independent thought. Everything in the human experience is connected through the ingredients of the biological matrix. Not only is this matrix a conduit for transforming and communicating, it is a living organism capable of producing original thoughts and responses to intentions and desires.

■ The Molecules of Emotion

The following examples illustrate the principle presented above. In her brilliant book, *Molecules of Emotion*, Candace Pert recounts the following story: Having read a groundbreaking paper on brain peptides in the immune system, she and a colleague, named Michael Ruff, set off to discover neuropeptide receptors in this system. A neuropeptide is a peptide that sometimes functions as a neurotransmitter. A peptide is any compound consisting of two or more amino acids. Amino acids are the building blocks of proteins. The union formed is called a "peptide bond." Peptides are combined to make proteins.

What they found was that every neuropeptide receptor they could find in the brain was also on the surface of a specialized form of white blood cell called the human monocyte. It identifies and digests foreign bodies. It is also responsible for wound healing and tissue-repair activity. They also found that the monocyte has receptors for peptide opiates, such as PCP. These substances, which affect emotions, also appear to control the routing and migration of the monocyte, which are central to the overall health of the organism. They also discovered that immune cells make the same chemicals that are associated with controlling mood in the brain. So, not only do immune cells govern the overall well-being of the tissues, they also manufacture chemicals that can regulate mood and/or emotion. This symbolizes the two-way communication between the brain and the body, which is a characteristic of the fundamental nature of the biochemical realm and the biological matrix.

■ More Than Just Molecules

Beyond the specific isolation of explicit substances that contribute to the function of the entire organism, subsequent interpretation leads us to suspect that the tissues, organs, and glands of the body are actually joined together in a sophisticated network of communication. Moreover, the evidence suggests that this interaction is bi-directional, supporting the assertion that the biochemistry is a transformational two-way thoroughfare of interaction. The same holds true for a host of other peptides and neuropeptides discovered in various systems of the body and the brain. The evidence continues to mount for a host of objective substances that exist locally and generally for the purposes of mediating specific function and maintaining wide-range communication throughout the body.

■ The Fields of Emotion

Dr. Pert demonstrated how neuropeptides, once thought to be only in the brain, are actually located in every cell in the body. She labeled these substances the molecules of emotion: "Our body is our subconscious mind and our mind is in our body, not just in our head, as is generally thought in our Western paradigm. The body is a field. Emotions are everywhere in the field and are triggered everywhere, therefore occurring in the head and the body at the same time. These molecules of emotion trigger different reactions and put the entire body in an altered state of consciousness doing what needs to be done in the moment, sometimes sleeping, emoting, excreting, etc." She describes how consciousness creates reality, and emotions are our link between the physical and spiritual. Her innovative research has produced volumes of similarly insightful revelations extolling the virtues of the biological matrix.

She writes: "Emotions are central to who we are as a person. They contribute to our interpersonal relationships, as well as the way we relate to ourselves. But we are living in a culture where emotions are suppressed. Just imagine the compensation that occurs as these unexpressed intentions accumulate. It is important to let our dynamic range be, and not restrict it so as to be stuck in any one pattern. It is this very process of inhibition that configures part of the foundation for habitual behavior." Not unlike Freud, Pert concludes that emotions are stored in the body and need to be dealt with in the body. We have better naturally occurring sources of neuropeptides than any drug or substance we can take from the outside. This potential predisposes us to be in a perpetually blissful state.

■ Chopra Meditation Experiment

In a less prominent, but no less significant, experiment, renowned healer and teacher, Deepak Chopra, describes the following experimentation. Several thousand people gathered for the purpose of meditating in a group environment. Each person in the group had their serotonin levels measured prior to the long meditation session. Serotonin is a neurotransmitter in the brain. Its presence in higher amounts is consistent with a feeling of calmness. The higher the serotonin level, the calmer and more peaceful you become. After several hours of group meditation, the levels of serotonin were measured again. There was a significant rise in these levels in practically all of the participants. The participants were all more peaceful and calm, consistent with the elevated serotonin levels.

However, there was a related feature to this experiment. It involved measuring the serotonin levels of people in the immediate vicinity of the meditation group who were not participating in the group meditation. Their serotonin levels were measured before and after the group meditation. The result was that simply being in the vicinity of those who were actually meditating significantly elevated the serotonin levels of those not participating in the meditation.

In yet another related experiment, Chopra associate, Cleve Baxter, developed a methodology for studying human cells that had been isolated from an individual body. In one experiment, he took human spermatozoa and studied them in a test tube to which he had attached an electrode. He was measuring their electromagnetic activity using a form of EEG instrumentation. The sperm donor was located about forty feet away in another room. When the sperm donor crushed a capsule of amyl nitrate and inhaled the fumes, there was an instantaneous spike in the electromagnetic activity of the test tube sperm rooms away.

In a related experiment, Baxter isolated white cells. Gold wires were connected to the EEG instrument and inserted into the white cells spun from his saliva. Simultaneously, he decided to inflict a cut on the back of his own hand and observe the activity of the white cells. After searching for a sterile lancet, he returned to induce the cut and noted that the electromagnetic activity of the cell sample had already increased in response to his intention to perform the procedure. These are but a few examples of well documented, but little known, experiments designed to substantiate the biocommunication of the human organism.

■ Self-Experiments

You can perform similar experiments on your own. Observe for a moment the universe around you. Now simply become aware. Direct your attention to some event, some phenomena, or some thought of your choosing. Begin to imagine what is already occurring in the world that envelops you and the world that you envelop. Envision two animals communicating through the transfer of a single molecule in the atmosphere called pheromones. Recognize the constant interchange of unspoken dialogue that occurs in your life each day as you interact with unspoken gestures, facial expressions, and gut feelings. Become aware of your body temperature and the changes that occur. Think about the urges you respond to daily. Remember the last time you felt physical pain. Bring to mind how you felt the last time you had a good night's sleep. Recall how you felt while you were last sleeping.

All of these things and more are examples of the intelligent universe enveloping us in every moment of our existence. If you truly stop for a moment to discover all of the amazing miracles occurring spontaneously within the borders of your unprompted awareness, you will have no doubt about your ability to create the reality of your dreams. Traversing the biological matrix into the realm of virtual authenticity, we approach the source of conscious creation. But before departing the river of biochemistry, disembark for just a few more minutes to explore some related features and events taking place simultaneously outside of conscious perception.

■ Applied Rorschach

Think of this experiment as a reflective Rorschach experience. Swiss psychiatrist Hermann Rorschach first introduced his famous inkblot pictures in 1921 as a form of analysis whereby patients looked at pictures and described what first came to mind. The results were characterized as a form of kinesthetic imagery whereby the images provoked a visual response and individual interpretation based upon subconscious associations. Instead of looking at pictures and describing what comes to mind, a form of word association using nothing but imagination will be employed. Instead of saying the words, simply think them and observe what comes to mind. Be aware of what you feel. Imagine how you feel it, and how your feelings change with each word. See where your imagination takes you.

Here is our list of words: Lemon, taxes, emergency, fall, cut, bruise, indigestion, rose, death, lottery, mother, Jamaica, iodine, sailboat, mucous, ammonia, blue, zero, work, void, love, juice, traffic, sand, mist, Disneyland, airplane, ambulance, lonely, laundry, chaos, cancer, Christmas, concert, ulcer, spa, massage, blond, water, pimple, sleep, news, math, memories, Italy, doctor, despair, angel, gift, weekend, ocean, snow, summer, grapes, fireworks, freeway, oysters, shopping, night, breeze, oxygen, cattle, church, gray, clouds, a part, apart, nowhere, now here, infinite, chainsaw, worms, mustard, God. Of course this list could on indefinitely. Any list can be created as a technique to assist in flushing out the subconscious and exploring stored-away impressions. While looking at these words, most people experience more than just the image reflected by the word. These words appear to trigger a cascade of thoughts, feelings, memories and emotions unique to their experiences. All of these encounters are integrated into who you are on every level. They are mediated through your biochemistry as the senses initiate the process of accessing stored information. This information is processed from a state of archived energy into electrical and biochemical intermediates that provoke attention to forgotten stimuli.

■ Who Are You?

The input that has become part of who you are is shaped with your participation into a cognitive experience. If your prefer a more simplified look at all that's been metabolized over the years, just take a look in the mirror. Step outside your thoughts, senses, emotions, feelings, imaginings, and memories. Just look! The virtual realm is where we experience the union of subjective and objective reality. It is in this realm that reality is created. It is in this realm that we can choose to willfully enact a specific and predictable outcome.

   With one foot in each of the tangible and intangible realms, constantly deciding which master to serve, Einstein's words silently shout, "Nothing happens until something moves." Movement is life. But will it be the foot or the thought that first moves the foot? Is it thinking that makes it like this? And if so, what moves the thought that moves? While these are all fascinating questions to ponder, they don't necessarily provide any tangible or practical tools for exercising anything but imagination. Not that that's a bad thing, but conscious participation in the process of creating our own life is the goal.

   Stimulating imagination (moving something) can provide motivation, inspiration, encouragement, and entertainment. However, movement for the sake of movement does not inevitably produce sustained momentum or a foundation upon which to create a new reality; that is, unless you've chosen to function exclusively in your imaginings. Unless you have, you will probably want to move on to more practical issues dealing with understanding the dynamics of the realms and your relationship to them.

A quick look back on the river just traversed provides further insight into some of the more obscure interactions that occur near the junction of the biochemical and the virtual realms. Keep in mind that swirling about within the confines of material reality are some more practical and mundane activities. One of the more accessible and most important activities is that of digestion.

■ CHAPTER SIX ■

The Question
of Digestion

"He that takes medicine and neglects diet, wastes the skill of the
physician."

—CHINESE PROVERB

Up to this point, I've touched on some practical and some interesting
characteristics of the biochemical world. But there are also some
options available for directly interacting with one's own biochemistry.
Let's step back from the minutia of the biochemical realm for a moment
and examine some fundamental events that relate to everyday performance.

The pH level (acid/alkaline measurement) of our internal fluids affects
every cell in our bodies. Extended acid imbalances of any kind can over-
whelm your body and interfere with normal function. When the pH of the
body gets out of balance (too acidic), we may experience low energy, fatigue,
excess weight, poor digestion, aches and pains, and even more serious disorders. Just as the body rigidly regulates its temperature, so will it attempt to

preserve a very narrow pH range—especially in the blood. The body will go to such great lengths to maintain a blood pH of 7.365 that it will even create stress on other systems to do so. Chronic acidification will interfere with all cellular activities and functions. As a result, it can interfere with life itself. Most people consume an abundance of highly processed foods that acidify the body. As a result, they are afflicted with many disorders that may be related, such as chronic fatigue syndrome, eczema, and ulcers.

On a very basic level, the body is an acid-producing machine. As the body engages in its daily encounters with all of the physical, biochemical, and virtual occurrences, it responds and changes in reply. On a gross biochemical level, these changes involve producing a metabolic waste product in the form of an acid. The body is designed to produce and eliminate this acid on a twenty-four-hour cycle. If more acid is produced than can be eliminated, it must be stored. Since acid is by nature corrosive, the body must create and retain buffers to neutralize the stored acid until it can be eliminated. How much buffering takes place depends upon how much acid is produced over what period of time, and how effectively it is eliminated. These same factors will determine what source of raw materials is used in the buffering process.

■ Buffering Acid Waste

Initially, most buffering is performed by oxygen. The body begins this buffering process by increasing the oxygen-binding capacity of the hemoglobin. This means that more oxygen is bound to the hemoglobin molecule within the red blood cells. This makes the oxygen unavailable for use on a cellular level. Initially, this has little, if any, effect on cellular buffering or energy production. However, over a long period of time, both functions are compromised. Before this compromise escalates to the point of irreversible damage, the body wisely shifts to another source of buffers. It turns next to the mineral supplies of the diet. The only potential obstacle at this juncture is the availability of minerals.

Here's how they translate to buffering: If the nutrients are not

Sources of Acidity

- Acidic diet.
- Toxicity and microform overgrowth.
- Improper elimination and neutralization of acids.

in the soil, they're not in the food. If they're not in the food, they're not in the diet. If they're not in the diet, they're not in the body. If they're not in the body, then another source has to be accessed. Inevitably, this source is bone. Subsequently, calcium and phosphorous are extracted from the bone to be used as emergency buffering resources.

Sound familiar? Is it possible that the true cause of the "diagnosable disease" known as osteoporosis is actually an excess acid burden stored in the body? Obviously, this is a subject of debate, but from my personal experience, I have seen tremendous increases in bone density occur by simply assisting the body in the removal of the stored acid burdens.

The process of restoring pH balance begins with proper diet and nutrition. This includes eating alkalizing foods, such as vegetables, low sugar fruits, etc., super hydration with alkaline water, and proper supplementation.

A practical diet plan for restoring the acid-alkaline balance of your body is the first step in reducing the acid burden. To operate in optimum health, our body needs balanced quantities of alkaline substances and acids. A chronic imbalance can result in health problems ranging from minor skin irritations, fibromyalgia, back pain, and depression, to arthritis, ulcers, and osteoporosis.

There is no need to organize alkaline and acidic foods on the basis of their chemical composition. A more effective approach categorizes foods based on their actual alkalizing or acidifying effect on the body. Some foods, such as fruits, can have either an alkalizing or an acidifying effect, depending on your own individual needs. Specific supplementation with alkaline supplements can support your dietary needs and goals, while assisting the body to remove excess acidic burdens that have accumulated over a long period of time. A complete system that combats acidity and its negative impact can be developed with the assitance of a Matrix Assessment Profile (M.A.P.), which we will discuss shortly.

■ And the Question Is?

Another issue related to mineral availability is the ability to access nutrients from our diet. If organically intact food sources are consumed and/or high quality minerals are supplemented, but digestion, absorption, and utilization are impaired, these meticulous efforts may be sorely compromised. Moreover, the question remains, what caused the inability to digest, absorb, and utilize properly? Was it the fundamental lack of raw materials to fuel the system, or was it the acid burden? If it was the acid burden, what caused it? Was it the lack of buffering materials, the inability to remove waste efficiently, or over exposure to acid-producing events?

■ The Essence of Digestion

To fully appreciate the dynamics of these issues, a basic understanding of digestion is essential. Although the details may be a little overwhelming, it is easy to see how the various systems within this arena contribute to orchestrating all of the biochemical events in the body. With an abundance of solid evidence linking digestive disease with shortened lifespan, illness, and lowered resistance to stress of all types, choosing a dietary format that works is one of the most important decisions we can make. But is that really enough?

Enzymes are essential to the efficient function of the entire digestive system. The environment in which these vital elements operate is equally important. Each phase of digestion plays a significant role in the overall process. One of the most important aspects of the process is the initial phase of stomach digestion. This phase has an intricate relationship to the second nervous system I discussed earlier.

From the mouth to the stomach, hormones begin to come into play. Preliminary versions of digestive enzymes are released in inactive forms to prevent the body from digesting itself. Their conversion to active status requires other enzymes called coenzymes. These coenzymes are dependent upon zinc and manganese. Deficiencies can result in digestive disturbances.

The acidity of the stomach may denature or render food enzymes ineffective. This suggests that animal-derived enzymes, such as chymotrypsin or trypsin, may be more effective in promoting optimal ingestion than their less stable vegetable counterparts, papain and bromelain. Following a brief period of time in the stomach, partially digested food is pushed by muscle contraction into the initial portion of the small intestine called the duodenum. Here, the intestinal phase of digestion continues, while a similar process takes place at each step in the sequence. Every phase has unique requirements involving enzymes, hormones, coenzymes, trace minerals, amino acids, and proper pH. Yet no focus is placed on ensuring that whatever is being taken in is also being digested and absorbed. The assumption is made that we all digest equally and completely.

A well-rounded wellness program must be based upon three simple concepts. Step one is to ensure the proper digestion of the proteins, carbohydrates, and fats necessary for the body to sustain health and vitality. Step two is to ensure adequate blood circulation for the proper transport of nutrients, hormones, white blood cells, etc., and for the timely removal of wastes. Step three provides for the maintenance of a good micro-flora within the gastrointestinal tract, which is an integral part of the body's biochemical, homeostatic, and immune systems. The bottom line is, we must give the body the nutrients it needs and clear away the waste.

■ Basic Requirements for Optimal Health

The biochemical environment comprises a full one-third of the human physical experience. Undeniably, it provides for a dynamic unseen substrate of activity. This activity contributes to every vital function, from reproduction to immune system response and repair. Complex in its overriding influence, the realm of nutritional biochemistry is reasonably simplistic in essence.

The human body has specific requirements that must be met on a daily basis to ensure optimal function. Theoretically, these requirements are to be met from the daily intake of food, beverages, water, and air. Additional requirements are then dictated by the activities of daily living. Long-term disruptions in the baseline quantity and quality of these supply systems leave the body to rely heavily on its ability to compensate under less than optimal circumstances. This is the situation in which genetic tendencies and nutrient deficiencies begin to demonstrate symptoms. Prolonged imbalances in these basic areas give rise to complicated symptom complexes that are rooted in the body's attempt to normalize through counterbalancing.

Part of this gradual accumulation of symptoms hinges on the ability of the body to compensate. To do this, it must first prioritize the distribution of nutrients based upon supply and demand. Substitutions are made, and nutrients are robbed from more abundant stores to maintain vital functions. Sacrifices are made to carry on economical function of the most critical systems. As additional compromises develop, these once low-grade imbalances begin to intensify into chronic distortions. All too often, these early symptom complexes are ignored as normal processes of aging and remain undetectable by conventional assessment. More often than not, these symptom complexes are permitted to accumulate until they take on a life of their own and appear to be a primary imbalance or even a diagnosable disease. In reality, they are just a reflection of the actual imbalance that produced them. Treatment amounts to simply treating symptoms and merely contributes to premature aging and death, while the underlying cause remains illusive and undetected.

■ Two Categories of Imbalance

Imbalances fall into two distinct categories. One is primary and predicated upon the actual deficiency or functional disturbance. Left undetected, it evolves into a pattern of more obscure symptom complexes. An example of a primary imbalance in the physical realm is that of headaches produced by pressure on a nerve due to contracted muscles following an automobile accident. In the biochemical realm, a primary imbalance might be that of frequent bruising caused by a bioflavanoid deficiency as a result of a lack of fresh fruits and vegetables in the diet. A primary imbalance in the virtual realm might be represented by the symptom of insomnia produced by excessive exposure to stress, or an inability to manage the long-term exposure to the stress.

The other category of imbalance is the compensated imbalance. It can actually present itself as a recognizable disease entity that may be unrelated to the actual imbalance from which it emerged. Examples of these might be the physical symptom of headaches produced by an inability to express emotions, or aberrant behaviors precipitated by diet-related chemical imbalances, environmental pollutants, or abusive relationships. The compensation occurs as the primary systems being stressed can no longer manage the assault associated with the stressing agent and distorts it in an attempt to maintain some form of homeostasis or balance. The resulting symptoms will then appear in a system that may be functionally related but entirely removed from the source of the actual stress, thus creating the illusion that the symptoms are originating in the system in which they appear. This is a very common occurrence when dealing with long-term biochemical imbalances that attempt to express themselves with physical symptoms, such as headaches, indigestion, gas, bloating, skin lesions, joint pain, and the like.

■ Reasonable Solutions

With the exception of a recently discovered substance that may increase the number of receptors associated with various addictions, evidently there is nothing that can be done about what we inherit genetically. However, reasonable precautions can be taken to avoid people, places, and things that have the propensity to increase risk and aggravate tendencies to express symptoms in this or any system. But is there anything that can be done other than designing a lifestyle around avoidance? Yes, yes, yes! Informed proactive choices are fundamental tools for ensuring optimal health and well-being. In the case of diet-related issues, supplements are indispensable.

■ Supplements Are Essential

Because of the current state of environmental affairs on our planet, five specific groups of nutrients must be supplemented on a daily basis. These include a broad spectrum multiple vitamin, a comprehensive mineral complex, an antioxidant, a probiotic and a digestive enzyme. The first and most important of these essential nutrients is the enzyme. Nowhere is this need for supplementation more critically evident than in the enzyme pools that provide the source for all repair and development in the body. Enzymes transform the ingested nutrients into vital functions allowing for the regeneration of blood, nerves, organs, and tissues.

■ Three Major Groups of Enzymes

Of the three major groups of enzymes, two are digestive and one is considered metabolic. Metabolic enzymes structure the basic elements of nutrition to be used by the body for its most vital functions. While metabolic enzymes are responsible for hormone production and development, they are also the single most important factor required to maintain a state of optimal well-being. They also provide the basis for a functional cure of diseases. It is also widely believed that enzyme activity governs the process of aging and determines the vitality expressed at any age.

Food enzymes initiate the process of digestion, while digestive enzymes continue the process of breaking nutrients down into particles small enough to be used by all of the systems of the body. Metabolic enzymes become active in the process of structuring these nutrients into nerves, organs, tissues, and blood. Optimally, enzyme stores will be replenished from food sources. However, in this modern technologically advanced society, it is unfortunately no longer feasible.

■ Enzyme Destruction

Any food heated above 118 degrees destroys all enzyme activity. Common cooking practices, processing, pasteurizing, blanching, irradiating and preservation leave little more enzyme activity than exists on a raw salad. Unfortunately, the general rule is that anything low in protein is usually low in enzymes. Salads are low in protein. The bottom line is that usable enzymes exist in only about 10 percent of the foods now available. But enzymes are needed in every bite of ingested food. Add to this the common practice of drinking carbonated beverages and taking antacids (two grossly overused patterns of behavior that also destroy enzyme activity), and it's amazing that our life expectancy is as long as it is. Quality of life is another issue altogether.

Why then, does life continue if the foods can't be digested without enzymes? Here's the rub! While eating raw foods, the teeth crush food cells, which release enzymes to assist in the process of digestion. Eating cooked food triggers mechanisms within the body that attempt to produce enzymes from their own resources. The pancreas is a major source of this activity. The raw materials for this process must now come from another source, since they are unavailable in the food itself. Therefore, the body must rob from the building blocks designated for the production of metabolic enzymes. The supply of enzyme materials is limited, and the body must now decide how to distribute what is available to accomplish the tasks of highest priority. At this moment, it is the digestion of the last ingested meal. So, what happens next? As this process continues throughout life, the body continues to rob from these finite stores to assist in a process that has been compromised as a result of modern technology.

■ Adapt and Compensate

The bottom line is that enzymes are needed. The body reallocates resources assigned to life-sustaining functions to permit the immediate process of digestion to continue. With the enzymes vacant from food sources, the body begins to compensate and adapt. No problem? No way! While the process of adaptation may not be evident in the earlier years of life, the faster the resources earmarked for the production of metabolic enzymes become depleted, the faster the aging process is accelerated. With this comes the hastened compensation of other vital functions. The pancreas swells, the brains shrinks, and life-sustaining processes are compromised until the body can no longer compensate. The early warning signs of disease are exhibited. Left unnoticed and unchecked, the ultimate result can be a diagnosable disease.

Hypothetically, eating an entire diet of raw organic foods will sufficiently address the potential depletion of enzymes. It may also provide the raw materials needed to maintain optimal biological function. Practically, however, it is difficult for the average person in this society to avoid cooked or processed food sources, let alone the stress, fear, anger, drugs, toxins, and pathogens that also inhibit the effectiveness of the enzyme systems. Realistically, the option is to supplement enzyme pools with a full complex of enzymes to assist in breaking foods down into usable components.

■ Enzyme Deficiency Warning Signs

Finally, the early warning signs of enzyme deficiency must be considered. These include symptoms such as frequent bloating, flatulence, and burping. Other symptoms may be as simple as fatigue and lethargy after eating, constipation, gas, stomach cramps, various food allergies, and susceptibility to frequent infections. Other more advanced symptoms may include mood swings, delayed wound healing, muscle wasting, skin problems, and diminished immunity.

We are not what we eat, but what we digest and absorb. Optimal well-being is dependent upon eating high-quality foods, proper digestion, absorption, distribution of nutrients, and elimination of waste. The process of digestion begins in the mouth and continues down through the stomach, pancreas, small intestine, liver, and gall bladder. Specialized processes occur at each step along this digestive pathway.

■ Critical Proteins

With an optimal diet in place, the process of breaking down these food materials into smaller particles and absorbing them is the responsibility of enzymes secreted in the digestive tract. Without enzymes, nothing happens. No energy can be produced, no food can be digested, and no nutrients can be absorbed. Vitamins, minerals, and hormones can do nothing in the absence of enzymes.

Each enzyme has a specific function and is specific to a particular food category. For example, enzymes called proteases break down proteins. Carbohydrates are broken down by amylases, while fats are degraded by lipases. Deficiencies in each of these specialized enzymes produce specific imbalances leading to predictable disease processes. For example, a protease deficiency will compromise the immune system, leaving the individual susceptible to frequent and recurrent infections. Fluid retention and toxic bowel syndrome are two other results of an inability to digest protein. Various intestinal problems, such as constipation, irritable bowel syndrome, appendicitis, and even colon cancer, have been associated with chronic protease deficiencies.

Meanwhile, incomplete protein digestion frequently results in low blood sugar and the associated symptoms of depression, irritability, and mood swings, as the sugar from protein metabolism is not available. Each deficient enzyme is capable of producing a wide assortment of common disease entities. These can include muscle soreness, asthma, altered insulin metabolism, elevated cholesterol, elevated triglycerides, and high blood pressure.

When an enzyme lack or deficiency exists, the food category dependent upon that enzyme does not get digested or absorbed properly. The result is intolerance to that food group. The biochemical foundation is then laid for specific disease processes associated with that particular deficiency. Intolerance to a particular food simply means that a particular food is not being digested properly. This is commonly associated with an enzyme imbalance or deficiency. Left unidentified and/or untreated, this enzyme discrepancy will demonstrate specific symptoms leading to predictable health problems.

In light of these simple facts, it is easy to understand why eight out of the top ten causes of death are directly related to diet, and why over 70 million Americans suffer from digestive problems, which lead to nearly 200,000 deaths each year. A troublesome issue now worth exploring is the byproduct of enzyme impairment—free radicals.

■ Free Radicals and Antioxidants

When ingested foods are incompletely broken down into their constituent components, a substance known as a free radical is formed. While this process is only one potential source of these toxic waste materials, it is extremely common and highly preventable by the simple addition of enzyme supplements to the diet. Free radicals are atoms or groups of atoms with an odd (unpaired) number of electrons and can be formed when oxygen interacts with certain molecules. Once formed, these highly reactive radicals can start a chain reaction like dominoes. The chief danger comes from the damage they can do when they react with important cellular components, such as DNA or the cell membrane. Cells may function poorly or die if this occurs.

To prevent free radical damage, the body has a defense system of substances known as antioxidants. Antioxidants are molecules that can safely interact with free radicals and terminate the chain reaction before vital molecules are damaged. Although there are several enzyme systems within the body that scavenge free radicals, the principle nutrient sources of antioxidants are vitamin E, beta-carotene, and vitamin C. Additionally, a trace mineral called selenium, which is required for the proper function of one antioxidant enzyme system, is sometimes included in this category. The body cannot manufacture these micronutrients, so they must be supplied in the diet.

■ Using Diet to Assist in Restoring Balance

Imperfect as contemporary dietary choices may be, there are some reliable approaches you can use to assure that your food preferences supply a reasonable nutrient base. Introducing an alkaline ash diet can replenish the dietary sources of alkaline reserve nutrients. By and large, these are mostly raw, organic foods that are rich in trace minerals, antioxidants, and enzymes. In general, most grains, dairy products, meats, seeds, legumes and nuts tend to have an acid ash. Most fruits and vegetables tend to have an alkaline ash. Foods such as orange juice and lemon juice are acidic but turn alkaline after they have been metabolized in the body. As such, for dietetic purposes, they are usually considered to be alkaline, despite being acidic prior to consumption. Most fruits are alkaline, except a few such as cranberries, plums and prunes, because they contain acids the body can't metabolize.

The purpose of an alkaline ash diet is to cause a fundamental alkaline shift in bodily fluids. This helps to create a productive environment for all of the body's metabolic processes. It also assists with any accumulated acid burden. Simultaneously, the tissues can be resaturated with supplemental trace minerals, while attempting to neutralize excess free radicals. This is accomplished with multiple individual nutrients designed to provoke a specific biological response.

■ The Environment Is Everything

The types of biochemical environments that allow for susceptibility to certain disease processes are well known. Also known are the types of internal environments that permit certain disease processes to proliferate. For these reasons, a baseline assessment at this level can prove invaluable in attempting to establish the biological wellness of an individual. If these environments can be effectively identified, potential disease processes can be isolated in the process of developing, prior to the appearance of a diagnosable disease. Comprehensive nutritional testing is an indispensable complement to conventional assessments, especially when dealing with undiagnosed symptoms.

The current medical literature is replete with information suggesting that illness develops in response to altered biochemical environments. Most recently touted are the dangerous implications of something as seemingly simple as an acid cellular environment. Recent observations indicate that this environment has been shown to be associated with the proliferation of such nemeses as viruses, parasites, mycobacterium, funguses, and even cancer cells.

In the early days of preventive healthcare, the assessment options were limited. Meticulous, time consuming, expensive, and labor-intensive methodologies were all that were available for identifying potential problems, and for developing a specific protocol for restoring balance to these delicate biological systems. During this time, programs were developed that involved severe dietary changes coupled with the inclusion of specific, but extreme, biochemical substances. These substances were capable of reversing the biochemical aberrations caused in the biological matrix by imbalances and deficiencies. Since then, technological advancements have streamlined this entire process for the patient and the practitioner.

■ Self-Help Can Help

A simple self-evaluation can be performed to determine the immediate or potential need for enzyme supplementation. Any individual can perform a cursory assessment of their own current needs by examining a few simple areas of their lives.

When performing a comprehensive self-evaluation begin with one of the caveats: "When you hear hoof beats, look for horses." First, look at the obvious—what foods and drinks are regularly consumed? Does the diet consist of primarily cooked or processed foods? This includes foods that are heated to temperatures of 118 degrees or above. Consider the current methods of cooking and preserving foods, such as blanching, boiling, microwaving, baking, and homogenizing, when making this assessment.

Next, consider the effects of fluids on digestion. Research suggests that for optimal digestion to occur, one or two glasses of room temperature water with a meal is essential for stimulating gastric, pancreatic, and intestinal responses. Carbonated beverages, or beverages that are excessively cooled, will inhibit these processes, as will excessive ingestion of coffee or alcohol. Then, consider the less obvious in the form of the daily environment in which you function. Evaluate your daily levels of exposure to air, food types (i.e., types and quantities of protein, carbohydrates, and fats). Also, take a look at the acid-producing potential of the foods you ingest, such as meats, citrus fruits, or acidic vegetables.

Don't forget to consider the additional exposures to excessive stress, emotional upset, medications, antacids, acid blockers, antibiotics, laxatives, birth control pills, fasting and herbs. This is essentially an opportunity for you to assess and communicate lifestyle beliefs and choices. It can be an invaluable tool when combined with pertinent history, clinical examination, and additional testing. We'll talk more about the appropriate types of testing in a moment.

■ The Ins and Outs of Nutritional Testing

So how does one know when nutritional testing is appropriate, and how does one know if what's being seen in the biochemistry is a cause or an effect? By definition, true nutritional testing incorporates an evaluation of the biochemical mechanisms that control, contribute to, and facilitate all of the activities that occur in the human body. Samples of blood, urine, and saliva are processed and evaluated to determine whether a productive biochemical environment exists. Assessment of primary activity levels will generally include pH, free radical activity, nutrient density, digestive function, energy production, elimination efficiency, detoxification capacity, and toxic burden accumulation. These parameters will then provide insight into related functions, such as immunity, heavy metal burdens, susceptibility, stress burdens, and specific organ integrity. Appropriate dietary and supplement recommendations can then be implemented based on the biochemical uniqueness of the individual.

The use of nutritional testing simplifies the process of identifying what we are seeing in the body as a cause or effect. Typically, individuals who subscribe to this type of testing fall into two categories. The first is the prevention-minded advocate. These individuals want to do everything they can to optimize function. They are interested in longevity and quality of life. The other group is much more widespread. They are individuals with unresolved symptoms, who have been everywhere and done everything, with no significant results. They simply want answers, and for the most part, just want to feel better. They want their symptoms to go away.

■ Two Main Types of Testing

At this point, it is simply important to recognize that there are two distinct categories of tests to choose from when assessing human biochemical function. The first category is that of the conventional assessment. This group of organized data is simply a set of tools agreed upon over time by individuals considered to be experts in this form of analysis. The tools are designed to assist in labeling an active disease process once it has been identified. These tools are relatively sophisticated, considering those available just fifty years ago, however they are far from being the most refined in existence. Typically, they rely on a conventional baseline arbitrarily established to differentiate a positive from negative test. In theory, a positive objective finding confirms the presence of the associated disease process and dictates treatment options.

The second category includes a group of tests designed to identify patterns of dysfunction that are in the process of developing into diagnosable disease entities. The concept here is that if a pattern of dysfunction can be associated with a known outcome, the outcome can be prevented. In the case of an individual who has endured subtle symptoms to the point of the expression of a diagnosable disease, the first group of tests is certainly helpful in prescribing a conventional course of treatment. However, it does little to assist in addressing the cause of the problem or to suggest viable treatment options. For the individual interested in prevention, or who suffers from chronic, low-grade, unidentified symptoms, the second group of tests is probably more effective and relevant.

■ The Magic of M.A.P.

M.A.P. is an acronym for Matrix Assessment Profile. While a comprehensive history is the cornerstone for this evaluation, a biological fluid analysis is the heart of the assessment. The process of transforming the biological matrix begins with a M.A.P. It provides an objective biochemical baseline for identifying the strengths, weaknesses, and imbalances in the fluids comprising the internal environment of your body that reflect the integrity of lymph, urine, and saliva formation.

The characteristics and condition of the fluids that compose this biological matrix may affect the entire body. This fluid matrix travels throughout the entire body, but each and every person is biologically and chemically unique. Each individual's cellular environment responds differently to stress, change, health, and illness. It also responds differently to all the factors that affect cellular functioning, such as genetics, hereditary issues, physical, mental, emotional, spiritual, social, and environmental factors.

In addition to assessing the relationship of these factors to your unresolved symptoms, a M.A.P. produces information specific to your biological environment regarding imbalances and deficiencies that may be potential causes related to your healthcare concerns. In short, a precise assessment and evaluation of the biological fluids may provide valuable information about underlying factors that may influence the overall state of your vitality and well-being.

The components assessed in this profile are used by the body to produce energy, to supply vital nutrients for sustaining life, and to create the biological fluids of urine, lymph, and saliva. Therefore, the chemical state of the biological matrix will be reflected in the results of the M.A.P. and provide a means of monitoring your response to therapeutic intervention.

Matrix transformation is the adapted science of evaluating and manipulating productive changes in the internal environment of the body. This environment is called the biological matrix. The biological matrix represents a fluid transport system for the delivery of nutrients to, and elimination of waste products from, the cells of the body.

The M.A.P. provides an assessment of the status of specific biochemical processes, which control and contribute to an ecologically competent organism. It also permits us a window of observation into this unique environment, allowing for invaluable insights into the ability of the cells to survive and prosper.

The M.A.P. assists in determining the physiological status of every major biological system in the body from two perspectives. First, it provides us with information pertaining to the three physiological factors of congestion, digestion, and energy production. Next it provides us with insight into how the body's glands, organs and physiological systems, such as the kidneys, liver, adrenals, digestion, elimination, etc., are being affected by association with the physiological factors.

With the latest advances in technology, the M.A.P. interpretation software is capable of determining similar values for the blood based upon the factors present in the other biological fluids. The use of this software allows us to offer the M.A.P. as a mail-order test. Now, anyone anywhere can have this testing done in the privacy of his or her own home and simply call to arrange for a convenient time to schedule a consultation. This makes the M.A.P. one of the most unique and comprehensive evaluations available.

The immediate goal of any approach designed to address a biochemical imbalance or deficiency is to assist the body in accessing its own nutrient pools. Secondary goals are to restore normal function and prevent the imbalance from reoccurring. There are a couple of steps in this process, and a couple of obstacles, to achieve a productive response, but the end results are highly achievable.

■ Other Benefits of Testing

Biochemistry represents a two-way bridge between the structural and virtual realms. Nutritional testing creates an access window into this viable channel of communication. The benefits of this type of testing go far beyond a simple biochemical assessment. It can actually help in establishing the realm of the primary imbalance and suggest effective approaches to resolving the associated symptoms.

For example, assume an individual goes to the doctor with any one of a group of common symptoms. Also assume that this individual has tested negative for any disease by all conventional standards. This is the profile of an individual with chronic, low-grade unresolved symptoms. For all intents and purposes, it is likely that it is not a structural problem and it probably isn't a diagnosable disease entity. Now what? Shall we wait and see? Should we suppress the symptoms? Should we send this person to a psychiatrist? Or perhaps nutritional testing might be a reasonable alternative.

Given everything presently known about the biochemical realm, nutritional testing would probably be a good place to start. There are a host of other possible tests that can be utilized to assess various biochemical aspects. Each of these has value (remember, everything works), however, some are more sensitive and specific to isolated issues, while others provide general information. With nutritional testing as a foundation, the appropriate inclusion of relevant tests can then be easily determined. As persistent symptoms remain unresolved and test results continue to return inconclusive or negative results, the more relevance many of these tests will have in differentiating the realm in which the causal imbalances are rooted. Generally speaking, the more enduring the symptoms and unfruitful the test results, the closer the probability of an imbalance rooted in the virtual realm.

■ Obstacles to Restoring Function

One of the potential obstacles in normalizing a chronically distorted biochemical environment is the loss of function. This loss occurs in conditions that have progressively deteriorated over a long period of time. In these cases, it is usually more realistic to aspire to management of the current state, while seeking to prevent further deterioration. All too frequently, an imbalance has progressed to a point where one of the following obstacles arise:

- The condition has been present for so long and the individual has tried so many things that he or she easily becomes frustrated and does not follow through.
- The identification of the probable cause stands in stark contrast to the wisdom of conventional assessments that brought the individual to seek alternative evaluations in the first place. Because of the seemingly simplistic, but far-fetched, potential solution to the problem, a half-hearted attempt fails to yield productive results.
- The major focus is on symptoms. While alteration of the biological matrix is consistent, it is also not instant. The symptoms do not improve fast enough for the patient to maintain participation.
- The individual with the imbalance lacks the discipline to follow through with all of the recommendations, and therefore fails to comply.
- Well-meaning friends and conventional practitioners who lack sufficient knowledge to support the endeavor discourage the individual with the imbalance.
- The program is time-consuming and costly.

■ Reality Check

Before breaching the threshold of a quantum lifestyle, a brief overview of some key concepts is necessary. Nutritional assessment is not limited to a dipstick acid test. It requires a sophisticated tool capable of establishing the status of the most critical biological parameters in the most viable bodily fluids. Overall, this assessment can aid in determining the status of everything from digestion to absorption, assimilation, utilization, and elimination in all the major systems of the body.

It is known that our soil has been severely trace mineral deficient for at least the last sixty years, and that approximately 80 percent of all degenerative disease has been linked to diet. It is evident that an assessment of this nature is vital in evaluating the true health status of any individual. The resulting findings are the indicators of an individual's unique biochemistry. This includes the current status and activities of enzymes, amino acids and other vital building blocks of life.

Generically, an altered biochemical matrix requires the inclusion of five specific groups of substances to achieve complete restoration and maintain the results achieved. These five substances include enzymes, probiotics (life-promoting bacteria), whole food vitamins, trace minerals, and antioxidants.

Supplements Are Critical

- Everyone must take five specific supplements daily: a broad spectrum multiple vitamin, a comprehensive mineral complex, an antioxidant, a probiotic and a digestive enzyme. Additional supplements are required on an individual basis.
- Nutritional testing is essential to developing a comprehensive program.
- Our biochemistry is a bi-directional link between the physical and the virtual.

The same intelligence that creates the body repairs and maintains the body. Symptoms are permitted to develop in an attempt to communicate the nature and extent of the imbalances that challenge the integrity of our life force. All too often, these attempts at communication are misinterpreted and seen as the problem.

Recent surveys indicate that 75–90 percent of all visits to physician offices are related to stress. Since it has already been established that life is stress, it is essential to have the tools available for identifying the source of the stress. Nutritional testing for the chronic sufferer is a good place to start, especially with statistics indicating a link between chronic, degenerative disease and diet.

■ CHAPTER SEVEN ■

New Horizons

"The test of a first-rate intelligence is the ability to hold two opposed ideas in the mind at the same time, and still retain the ability to function."

—F. Scott Fitzgerald, U.S. novelist (1896–1940)

In attempting to eliminate an apparent disease, it is important to ask whether its true cause has been determined, or is it merely the symptoms of imbalance that allow for the expression of a diagnosable entity? What truly causes a person to become ill? Without a cause, how is a cure even possible? This is the current dilemma of conventional medical science. This is the frustrating reality facing researchers. Herein, lies the causal dynamic of Vicious Cycle Disorders. This is the motivation for considering the whole person before initiating any therapeutic intervention. This is the promise that lies beyond science and beyond medicine.

Given that the body is an amazing and miraculous piece of machinery, there's much more going on here than meets the eye. "Inside out," and "As above, so below," are simplistic analogies that convey wisdom beyond words. Yet, while observable, the innate wisdom of statements such as these is beyond the scrutiny of conventional scientific assessment. This wisdom also seems of little use in resolving the chronic symptoms of ailing patients. Or is it? Arguments persist on both sides of the debate as to whether it is more effective to treat the body through the mind, or the mind through the body. There is ample evidence to support both approaches.

One side of the bias holds that matter is dominant over mind. This school of thought asserts that there is no correlation between a state of mind and a disease process. Volumes of well-constructed studies at prestigious institutions confirm this position. Many are reported in prominent publications, such as the *New England Journal of Medicine.* By illustration, one such study performed in 1985 at the University of Pennsylvania concluded that disease, as a direct reflection of mental status, is largely folklore.

My personal opinion is that this study and other similar studies are basically flawed. I believe that these studies are merely designed to observe the effects of a contrived set of circumstances that are impossible to comprehend. These circumstances include the state of mind of the individual being observed. While possible to obtain some subjective data as to what the individual is thinking or feeling, it is impossible to know their thoughts. Remember that the best current estimate is 60,000 thoughts per day.

In the other camp, convincing research suggests something quite to the contrary. For instance, at my undergraduate alma mater, Ohio University, an unexpected finding was reported during a heart disease study in 1970. Highly toxic, high-cholesterol diets were fed to rabbits in an attempt to produce the blocked arteries associated with similar diets in humans. Findings in all the rabbit groups were consistent, except one. This one group displayed 60 percent fewer symptoms for no apparent reason. No apparent reason, that is, until an incidental finding was disclosed. It was discovered that this one group of rabbits was getting something that the other groups were not. They were being stroked and caressed by their caretaker prior to being fed. Repeat experiments produced similar results. This study, although a bit more holistic in nature, is actually substantially more valid. It actually documents an observable and reproducible response under controlled circumstances in which the variables are well known and established.

■ Mind-Body Science

Since the emergence of the various counterparts in the mind-body movement, numerous and more aggressive studies have emerged to support both sides of the issue. The blatant polarity of these positions ultimately goes to suggest that they are both part of a larger dynamic.

Nonetheless, the mind-body frontier is the research laboratory of the future. Simply asking someone how they feel at any given moment about a particular issue is entirely too subjective to substantiate a firm position regarding cause and effect. This shows the need for caveats to serve as guides through the process of determining cause to achieve a cure. Given the number of thoughts an individual may have in any given day, and the fact that this is occurring in billions of people who are constantly interacting, one can only observe the net effects of the interface. Because everyone affects, and is affected by, everything continually, reality based upon this fundamental exchange is variable at best.

If just one person experiences a spontaneous remission, it is proof enough that another dynamic is at work that just hasn't been identified yet. Sooner or later, the mechanism of cure will be quantified and refined. In fact, a detailed explanation for such a phenomenon has already been addressed in the world of quantum physics. Recalling our earlier discussion of probability and possibility, genetics is quantified probability. It is concerned with the statistical likelihood of something occurring. The more something happens, the more likely it is to occur again.

Meanwhile, just because something hasn't happened yet (or hasn't yet been observed), doesn't mean that it can't or won't happen. Therein, lies the unresolved mystery, and in the mystery, the solution. All the rest are stories about observations to support the reality of a personal belief system. In other words, the explanation, impression, or expressed opinion concerning a condition, group of unresolved symptoms, or unexplainable cure is presented within the context of what a given individual believes to be true. For instance, I have seen what might be called spontaneous remission in numerous patients over the years. By example, the cases that follow illustrate the unpredictability of the variables involved in a complete and total "restoration to health." They also embody a cause-specific "cure," and demonstrate the central point of the caveats.

■ Cause-Specific Cures

A forty-two-year-old female came to my office with concerns about hair loss. Upon examination, it was evident that she was losing hair in large clumps. No effort was required to extract the hair. It was practically falling out of her head. Needless to say, she was quite distraught over this occurrence.

Following an evaluation protocol that included a M.A.P., I determined a course of treatment to which she agreed and complied. Within three weeks, she was completely bald. Within four months of our initial encounter, however, a full head of hair more vibrant than her original had re-grown. She maintains it to this day. That was seven years ago from this writing.

Her causal complex demonstrated two obvious features. The first was extreme internalization of stress, accompanied by depression and anxiety. The second was repeated exposure to highly toxic environmental chemicals associated with her employment. Once the mechanisms within the system under stress were identified, a specific protocol was implemented to support a return to equilibrium. Shortly thereafter, her body's attempt to communicate through the symptom of hair loss was terminated.

Since the point of this example is not to suggest a cure for the symptom of hair loss, I will not detail the entire process. However this representation is a good example of the "everything works" and "hoof beats" caveats. I began with the obvious and searched for the most likely causes first. Her program was detailed and she began to respond. Despite the learned skill of internalizing stress, she was receptive, cooperative, and responsive. There was no denial here, only a lack of information.

■ Seizure Symptoms

Similarly, I was presented with an eighteen-month-old female infant who was born into a loving and caring family under normal circumstances. For the first twelve months of her life, everything was perfect. In her twelfth month, however, she began to develop seizures. Multiple opinions and evaluations later, her parents brought her to my office having twelve seizures per day. There was no organic source for the seizures, so she was diagnosed with idiopathic non-organic seizure disorder and medicated. The medications weren't helping and there appeared to be no hope for the stressed-out new parents.

With all of the conventional assessments being negative, I decided to look at the situation in a different way. I ran a series of alternative assessments. Thereafter, I developed a simple and conservative protocol and implemented it immediately. Despite some skepticism, they were desperate for help, so they religiously complied. Within two weeks, the child was symptom-free. No seizures! Within two months, she was off all medications and stable. She remains healthy, vibrant, and seizure-free to this day. Our original contact was nearly two years ago from this writing.

The protocol I followed to determine the course of treatment was consistent with the differential diagnosis format that I developed for VCD involving the caveats and the M.A.P. In this particular case, it was quickly evident that the child was suffering from a genetic tendency that expressed itself subsequent to specific physical and environmental stress factors. Her particular imbalance revolved around compromised digestive enzyme activity and gross trace mineral deficiencies. Once identified and addressed, her symptoms resolved immediately and have never returned.

Once again, this is not a dissertation on the treatment of seizure symptoms, but it does illustrate the power of cause-specific treatment. With the possible exception of hit-or-miss responses, the treatment, in and of itself, would be of no benefit to the seizure population at large.

■ Other Worldly Symptoms

By contrast, I encountered a fourteen-year-old female who had undergone a head and neck trauma while at school. Nine months after the incident and numerous approaches later, she came to my office. She was still wearing a hard neck brace and complaining of severe neck pain with headaches. She was also bent over looking at the floor. She indicated that the pain was so severe she could not stand upright. In addition, she was being fed through a tube because she could not eat solid food due to nausea and vomiting. She hadn't eaten solid food for nine months.

After reviewing her history and examining her, I determined that one of two possibilities existed. One was that the actual structural source of the injury had yet to be identified. It is possible for certain neurological structures to produce the symptoms she was experiencing. The other possibility was that she was suffering from a form of post-traumatic stress syndrome causing the autonomic nervous system to override the voluntary muscles of the body. This could cause a syndrome called somato-sensory amnesia. Due to the shock and trauma of the incident, her body shut down and forgot how to work.

As the next several months unfolded, the details of her care became more convoluted. In addition to the four or five hours per week in my office receiving conservative structural care, there were intermittent visits to the emergency room, ancillary evaluations by specialists, and multiple attempts to acquire more specific diagnostic information. Weeks turned into months, with more treatments, more tests, more doctor visits, and no response whatsoever. Because of the length of time since her injury, and the emerging stress on her internal organs from the external feedings, the concern mounted. Still no change was in sight. She now needed to be home schooled. Her condition continued to degenerate, with no hope in sight, and no additional evidence to support any obvious diagnosis. Road trips to out-of-town specialty hospitals proved equally fruitless. Child protective services became interested.

■ Virtual Reality

The ensuing dynamic was almost too strange to believe. Frustrations mounted, accusations flew freely, and this young girl was deteriorating rapidly. As I stepped back from the picture, my suspicions mounted. What began as an attempt to engage the girl's mother in a non-threatening discourse proved to be lethal to our relationship. As I breached the likelihood that another possibility existed in the virtual realm, a raw nerve became inflamed. They both stormed out of my office never to be seen or heard from again.

Without going into the family dynamics and the specifics of the various interactions occurring among those involved, it was obvious that something was very wrong. In fact, several months later my suspicions were confirmed. This entire drama had taken seed in the virtual realm and sprouted into the material world as a physical disability. Following the caveats through the process of differential diagnosis was cumbersome, and painful in this case. Nonetheless, it provided me with the roadmap required to ultimately resolve this child's dilemma. A true psycho-emotional-spiritual drama had unfolded right before my eyes.

Initially, the girl's situation was provoked by an acute physical trauma. However, as her condition progressed, it was evident that the physical trauma was merely an opportunity for some severely repressed emotional concerns to express themselves. This fact became more obvious as physical attempts to identify and treat the apparent cause proved futile. Simultaneously, the emotional climate escalated with each failed attempt and negative test result.

By the time I became involved in this drama, it had completely changed forms. Nonetheless, by process of elimination, I was able to isolate the cause to the virtual realm. Eventually, the teen was admitted to a prestigious facility where an intervention was performed. The realm in which the cause of her physical expression of impairment was rooted was isolated, identified and treated. I'm happy to say that the entire family received the help they needed and the youth has been returned to the upright position, eating solid food, and enjoying the privileges of driving, while exploring her teenage years as a healthy optimistic young lady.

In sharing these dissimilar stories, I reiterate my earlier point. The more something happens, the more likely it is to occur again. However, just because something hasn't happened yet (or we haven't yet observed it), doesn't mean that it can't or won't happen. Therein, lies the unresolved mystery, and in the mystery, the solution. All the rest are simply stories about observations to support the reality of a belief system. Sometimes the belief system is merely an agenda that represents a fundamental sense of entitlement on the part of the patient with the symptoms. They have somehow come to believe that they are at liberty to express behavior or receive attention through their physical ailment that has otherwise been denied them in other areas of their lives. Other times, the belief system is perpetuated by a healthcare professional that feels threatened by an inability to successfully resolve a patient's issue and expresses his or her insecurity through the dogmatic adherence to a condescending and self-righteous attitude or behavior. That being said, I am more convinced than ever that there can be no problem without a solution. The solution is always contained within the problem, however the problem is not always where or what it appears to be.

■ Abnormally Normal

The blatant polarity of the positions espoused by the opponents in the mind-body controversy ultimately goes to suggest support for the fact that they are both part of a grander scheme. After almost thirty years of seeing every imaginable symptom manifest itself in unpredictable and unusual ways, and similarly extraordinary cures, I am of the opinion that both sides are right. They're just not both right all the time. Hence the caveat "everything works." However, to achieve optimal results from the application of a given modality to a set of circumstances, the selection of tools must be specific and appropriate. In other words, to resolve a disruption of normal function, we must know the cause of the disruption and where the cause is rooted.

Having said that, there is a subcategory of patients who function well in mild degrees of imbalance. In these cases, it is difficult to identify a cause simply, since it exists in the mind of the patient experiencing the symptoms. These symptoms are typically chronic and low-grade. These symptoms also tend to involve all three realms, since an undisclosed need is being fulfilled by the functional imbalance. In other words, the patient is deriving some satisfaction from his or her apparent dysfunctional behavior. There is some payoff for perpetuating the imbalance that produces the symptoms.

Usually the symptoms are more pronounced than any objective findings. Any attempt to address cause is quickly thwarted by distractions. These typically arise in a realm other than the one being focused on for treatment. This is, by and large, a sure sign that one is on the right tract. However, efforts to shape a remedy are discouraged and resisted by the patient. If one persists in their efforts to encourage resolution, more times than not, the patient will discontinue care.

Meanwhile, these patients tend to be devoted to the point that a pseudo-dependency develops, along with enough cooperation to maintain the relationship. Generally, these individuals are harmless and simply experience some deep lack. This allows them to present themselves with just enough low-grade symptoms to feed their need through a relationship with a caring provider. Once identified, it becomes the choice of the caregiver as to whether or not to continue with the relationship. Nurtured over an extended period of time, these individuals tend to respond productively, albeit slowly.

Given the scenarios just presented, I am decidedly persuaded that there are no true diseases. Diagnosable diseases may simply be the end result of a much subtler process. Disease entities may be the outcome of an undiagnosed long-term imbalance seeking expression in the form of a last-ditch attempt to get our attention. These imbalances can originate in any of the three realms or through their by-products.

■ The Hammer and the Nail

In my previous book, *A Question of Balance*, I shared a story that aptly illustrates cause and effect in the physical realm. It is also a suitable example of the "hammer and nail" caveat. For this purpose, I would like to share it again here. Some time ago, I had the opportunity to evaluate the concerns of a young man who came to me with symptoms of pain in the left shoulder. Despite numerous attempts by a wide variety of healthcare professionals to eliminate his discomfort, it persisted and seemed unaffected by these efforts.

Prior to his reluctant appearance in my office, he had subjected himself to many of the usual, and some quite unusual, assessments and treatments for the symptom of shoulder pain. His pain was unyielding in its response to treatment. He continued to be passed along with the diagnosis of chronic shoulder pain. All of the treatments to date had been directed toward the site on his shoulder where the symptom of pain expressed itself. Physically, he seemed to be a healthy and robust young man with an interest in weightlifting. The symptoms had progressively worsened over a period of months. X-rays, MRI, orthopedic evaluations and diagnostic ultrasounds yielded no clue as to the source of the pain.

Cortisone injections, massages, and a wide variety of home therapies provided no relief. Despite the best-intentioned efforts of all the individuals he consulted for the problem, his shoulder pain persisted. He remained a victim of the hammer and nail syndrome. As you recall, this caveat dictates that when all you have is a hammer, everything looks like a nail. As I suggested earlier, one of the dilemmas of our specialized healthcare environment is that we all tend to evaluate and treat from the perspective of our specialized training.

Despite a broad-based foundation in differential diagnosis, an orthopedic surgeon might perceive the shoulder pain as a joint dysfunction. A chiropractor may view it as a spinal instability. A massage therapist might construe it as a muscle imbalance. An acupuncturist may see it as a meridian problem, while a psychotherapist may diagnose unexpressed anger. In reality, they may all be right to some extent. Unfortunately, none of them accurately reflects the causal mechanism that resulted in the expression of the specific symptoms.

The actual source of the imbalance was direct trauma to the subscapularis muscle. This is a small, frequently overlooked muscle that lies beneath the shoulder blade, i.e. scapulae. It was originally injured due to a combination of using too much weight in conjunction with poor technique, overstretching, and overuse. Repetitive micro-trauma accumulated into small trigger points as he continued to try and use the injured shoulder. This simply means that, at some point, he actually injured one of the muscles attached to the shoulder joint. The initial injury itself was so subtle that it went unnoticed until it escalated to the point that it affected his performance. To that point, he simply assumed it to be post-workout soreness.

As he continued to use it, scar tissue began to form. The circulation to the tissue was compromised. Nutrients could not be delivered and waste product could not be removed. So the metabolic waste became trapped in the tissue and caused inflammation. This reactive inflammation, once identified and neutralized, eliminated the shoulder pain during the course of his initial treatment utilizing a combination of moist heat, manipulation, and neuromuscular therapy. Superficially, this appears to be a tribute to astute diagnostic skills. However, it is illustrative of the potential inherent in the application of the caveats. If you look closely at this case history, you'll see all of the caveats present. Of course, there is the hammer and nail caveat. Not far behind is the hoof beats and horses caveat. This is followed closely by everything works, no panaceas, and the action/reaction caveat.

■ Everything Is What It Isn't

As observed in the previous example, the apparent shoulder pain was, in fact, pain in the shoulder. However, it was not shoulder pain per se. It was pain expressed as a result of an imbalance in the underlying musculature that presented itself as pain in the shoulder. A similar dilemma exists in a broader deliberation of cause and effect. In the case of expansive symptom complexes, the diagnosis is frequently a moot point. Too often, the temptation is to see the presenting symptom as the focus of well-intended efforts, rather than acknowledging the person who is exhibiting the symptoms of imbalance.

A whole person point of view presents the simple complexity of determining cause to determine effective treatment. This model can be simplified to represent the entire domain of human experience, as it obviously includes the physical, the biochemical and the psycho-emotional-spiritual (or virtual) realms of possibilities.

■ The Chicken and the Egg

Operating from this whole person model, the age-old "chicken and egg" metaphor can be aptly referenced. For centuries, a debate ensued among the great minds of the healing arts. The essence of this controversy revolved around the proposition that disease entities actually caused disease. For instance, a germ or virus would invade the body and advance an assault resulting in an ailment. Disease was thought to be organism-specific.

Opponents of this view held that disease agents were everywhere all the time, and merely took advantage of an opportunity to invade and subdue susceptible or diseased tissue. This would suggest that the various agents of doom were not the actual cause of the affliction. Rather, the nature of the diseased tissue was the determining factor that dictated the extent to which symptoms might express themselves.

On his deathbed, Louis Pasteur is reported to have yielded to this theory, suggesting that the terrain is everything. Despite this quiet acknowledgment, the "doctrine of specific cause" was adopted as a basis for the modern medical model. This theory asserts that a single microorganism is the sole causal factor in producing specific symptoms of disease in an otherwise healthy organism. The overall condition of the whole person was discarded in exchange for the single cause theory. Despite overwhelming evidence to the contrary, the millennium of the microscope unveiled detailed descriptive data for examining the effects of disease. It also abolished any consideration of the susceptible environment in which disease might propagate.

H.R. Holman, M.D., from Stanford University, aptly summarized this dilemma in his presentation on "the crisis in healthcare." He stated, "Some medical outcomes are inadequate not because appropriate technical interventions are lacking, but because our conceptual thinking is inadequate." Based upon this premise, we might assume that healthy tissue could be the ultimate defense against the ravages of foreign intruders. What causes or allows normal, healthy tissue to become compromised to the extent that it yields to these disease-generating trespassers? What can we do to prevent the ravages of age from becoming the source of an endless series of painful physical experiences resulting in disease and death? A consideration of the intrinsic nature of balance within each of the three realms is essential to fully grasp the latent potential in these questions. Since the realms embody the entirety of one's life experience, a closer look is central to an appreciation of their significance.

■ CHAPTER EIGHT ■

A Day in the Realm

"Every creator painfully experiences the chasm between his inner vision and its ultimate expression."

—ISAAC BASHEVIS SINGER, U.S. (POLISH-BORN) AUTHOR (1904–1991)

A s each realm attempts to preserve its natural balance, the relationship among the realms will ultimately express overall stability. This is true to the highest degree. However, another dynamic comes into play when the concept of counterbalance or compensation is considered. Looking at things differently, it becomes apparent that disease is not only the end result of a process, but is, in essence, the process. This allows for seeing not only what something is, but also what it isn't.

■ Classical Chiropractic

Take, for example, a simple scenario from the concept of classical chiropractic practice. This assertion is the common theme running throughout all chiropractic philosophy. The theme is that of a chronic subluxation of specific spinal segments causing dysfunction and disease. Subluxation generally refers to a misaligned bone of the spinal column. Ordinarily, when one thinks of a malpositioned vertebra, a related physical insult is implied as its cause. Oftentimes, this is true. Misalignments can be caused by physical trauma, repetitive movements, or prolonged positional stress. But here's the twist. The subluxation or misalignment in the example we are about to examine exists as a result of impaired carbohydrate digestion, not physical trauma.

The salivary glands, which are located in and around the mouth, receive a portion of their innervation (nerve supply) from an allotment of the autonomic or automatic aspect of the nervous system. These are known as sympathetic nerves. More specifically, this innervation arises from the first and second thoracic spinal nerves at the base of the neck. These nerves send branches through a series of nerve complexes up the neck to allow for signals to reach many muscles in the head and face. *All* the muscles of the neck, shoulders, and upper extremities are included in this complex.

Spinal nerves originate from the spinal cord and proceed to other structures in the body. At that point, they exert influence on the function of that structure and communicate information back through the spinal cord to the brain. The idea is that organ and/or tissue dysfunction (a form of stress) causes muscle contraction in the group of muscles that share a common spinal nerve supply with that tissue or organ. Therefore, it becomes possible, if not probable, that a chronic recurring pattern of dysfunction in the structures at this level of the spine may be receiving their stimulus as a result of a glandular dysfunction. In this case, the salivary gland's inability to perpetuate carbohydrate digestion, due to a lack of adequate nutrition, initiates the dysfunction. This results in the symptom of subluxation.

The gland, which is stressed in its attempt to perform its routine function, hypertrophies (enlarges) in an attempt to compensate for its lack of ability to perform normally. This hyperactivity results in hyper stimulation, which causes muscle contractions and subsequent lower neck pain. Treating the recurring neck pain without addressing the underlying cause of cellular malnutrition becomes as fruitless as the attempts to eliminate the shoulder pain (in our previous example) with cortisone injections. This concept exemplifies the view that imbalance within any one area will cause a related area to compensate by counterbalancing the effects. This is performed in an effort to maintain equilibrium within the entire system. It is also an attempt to communicate the imbalance with vague, recurrent symptoms.

■ Early Indicators of Developing Disease

Symptoms are the early indicators of a disease that has not progressed to the point of a diagnosable entity. At this stage, it is referred to as a subclinical imbalance. It is yet to be revealed, recognized or expressed as an actual disease. Herein, lie the beginnings of ultimate destruction. The potential of these seeds of imbalance is nurtured by repetitive patterns of behavior. These patterns support the development of diagnosable disease entities. This is the blueprint for the advancement of Vicious Cycle Disorders.

An everyday instance of this dynamic might be that of simple cravings. In general, these cravings may simply represent an early form of cellular malnutrition caused by a diet deficient in trace minerals. The deficiency originates as a consequence of our depleted soil not being replenished with the vital nutrients extracted during the process of cultivating crops for consumption. The result is that of nutritionally inadequate food sources being the intermediate cause of cravings. Often these cravings will be associated with addictive behavior syndromes. More often, they are misdiagnosed as a behavioral disorder, when in fact; they are merely symptoms of an underlying imbalance in a fundamental biochemical mechanism. This is an example of something being what it isn't. This is a behavioral disorder, however the behavior is a symptom of the underlying biochemical imbalance. The imbalance is the actual cause. When discovered (or looked at in this way) the appropriate treatment is more easily recognized.

In the previous example, I referred to something being what it isn't. This observation is not only a caveat, but also a characteristic of VCD. To be a true form of VCD, this characteristic must always be present. Although difficult to recognize initially, it will become more obvious as the cycle matures and becomes more dominant.

■ A New Model of Diagnosis

For the cause of vague and persistent symptoms to be detected in the absence of a diagnosable disease, a new model of differential diagnosis must emerge. The clinical challenge becomes that of determining which symptoms are associated with which cause. The goal is to restore balance to the whole person, rather than masking the emerging symptoms of an imbalance to create the illusion of balance.

Clinically, imbalances associated with VCD will present themselves as symptoms of commonly diagnosed ailments, such as obsessive compulsive and attention deficit disorders. All too frequently, the symptoms are diagnosed and treated as a disease. In reality, all that is accomplished is the artificial management of a group of symptoms. This only serves to perpetuate and aggravate the fundamental imbalance. The causes are overlooked simply because this aspect of the dynamic is frequently overlooked, if considered at all. With rare exceptions, a psychiatric opinion is requested.

The recent popularity of attention deficit hyperactivity disorders, and the subsequent prescription of Ritalin or other similar drugs, is a timely example of this mistreatment. Ritalin is a powerful drug with dangerous side effects. The common side effects include psychotic symptoms, depression, addiction and rebound dependency. Yet it is prescribed routinely for the disorders noted above. These disorders more commonly arise from a habitual and insidious addiction to refined sugar, as well as gross nutrient deficiencies. It is possible to restore equilibrium very quickly when this imbalance is looked at differently. Often, simply monitoring sugar intake and supplementing the diet with trace minerals, grape seed extract and multi-enzymes can improve or resolve these symptoms.

■ Two Attitudes, Two Solutions

In the example above, two solutions deal with different aspects of the same problem. One solution is directed toward the symptomatic relief of a biochemically imbalanced system. This is merely another example of something being what it isn't—a true solution. The other solution is directed toward eliminating the cause. As lifestyle dynamics are evaluated from this perspective, a practical fact is discovered. Healthcare can be approached with one of two attitudes. One is an outlook of prevention. From this perspective, the symptoms of disease are assessed as indicators of imbalance. From the other, the strategy is to wait until the imbalance becomes a diagnosable disease entity and then engage in crises intervention. This is known as disease management. It is a choice not only for the practitioner, but also for the person with the symptoms.

■ Functional Hypoadrenia

Another common example of an imbalance in one area causing the other systems to compensate is that of a condition known as functional hypoadrenia. In this example, a progressive series of imbalances produces a progressive series of symptoms that result in a diagnosable disease. These recurrent symptoms give rise to the false appearance of a disease. This false appearance and coincident misdiagnosis nurture an inevitable expression of fear of the unknown. In this case, the presence of fear illustrates the acronym made prominent by motivational speaker Zig Ziglar: F.alse E.vidence A.ppearing R.eal. The ultimate disease is merely the end result of an imbalance that was not identified and can no longer be compensated for by the system in which it originated. In actuality, functional hypoadrenia is a normal reaction within the body that occurs on a daily basis in response to what we perceive as stress. It is one of the few disorders that are actually self-perpetuating in that it produces more of itself.

Hans Selye, in his book, *The Stress Of Life*, illustrates the difficulty in defining this popular topic of literary and social discussion. The word "stress," like "success," "failure," or "happiness," means different things to different people. In the medical sense, stress is essentially the rate of wear and tear in the body. With the advent of more sophisticated diagnostic tools predicated upon the original work of Louis Pasteur and others, stress is this rate of wear translated into a biological age. Biological age is a theoretical number that suggests the rate at which our bodies are aging compared to our actual chronological age. It is based upon a variety of arbitrary parameters that accurately reflect this process of deterioration. It is often helpful as an adjunctive trait that can be monitored and managed to reflect the effectiveness of a given treatment approach.

■ Predictable Reactions

In my own clinical and personal experience, stress appears to be a reaction-producing reaction. This phenomenon includes a set of fairly predictable physiological reactions to any stimulus. Combined with some less predictable responses involving individual genetics, learning experiences, and tolerances, these reactions can prematurely advance the biological age.

The reaction-producing reaction is rooted in the priority system of the body. This system is designed to regulate our response to perceived stresses. Physiologically, the body does not differentiate the nature of the stress, nor its response to it. In an attempt to maintain harmony at all costs, the body merely reacts to the numerous balance-threatening stimuli encountered on a daily basis. This is known as homeostasis. Yet, individual responses to each stressing agent may be as unique as the individual stressor. This uniqueness determines whether stress will merely be experienced, or whether distress will manifest itself as a symptom of VCD. The stress of life includes all of the people, circumstances and events encountered on a daily basis. Stress is inherent in the quest for activity, fulfillment, and personal satisfaction. It can also be produced by chance encounters with resistant strains of viruses and bacteria, as well as unpredictable contact with other people going through their own individual life changes.

■ Life Is Stressful

It is interesting to note that stress is not produced just from things considered to be bad or harmful. Stress reactions are produced by the anticipation of seeing a long-lost friend or relative, the promise of intense pleasure, or the ecstasy of fulfillment. From this perspective, it may be assumed that everything is or has the capacity to produce stress. Thus, life is stress.

Discipline in the form of exercise, meditation, diet, and abstinence qualifies as a stressor, but so does indulgence to excess. This produces stress in related areas. In moderation, these stressors have the capability of being rejuvenating. They are filled with the potential for self-enhancement, again demonstrating that "everything is what it isn't." Looking more closely at some common examples, it is easy to see the unlimited possibilities for stress to be experienced and for distress to be manifested. Consider the occurrence of a simple itch on the arm. The initial response usually involves scratching it a couple of times to relieve the immediate physical discomfort. The stress is experienced and resolved. It is primarily a temporary physical experience at this stage.

However, when bombarded repetitively by inordinate amounts of what the body perceives as stress, a number of specific mechanisms are employed in reply. Observe this progression as a simple itch becomes more persistent. A more aggressive scratching is employed to subdue the itch, while adding some topical agent known to be effective in neutralizing such concerns. The body, on the other hand, initiates a first-stage response to the acute stress. This includes a flood of hormones from a portion of the adrenal glands called the medulla. This reaction, in turn, stimulates the body to engage the stress. Once this mechanism has been successful in neutralizing the stress, the body resumes its natural state of balance or homeostasis. Should the stress persist, the body proceeds into a more motivated effort to adapt. Additional hormones are secreted in an attempt to manage the source of the stress, rather than conquer it.

As the itch persists and develops into a chronic skin condition, long-term exposure to the stress depletes the ability of the body to adapt at this level. This results in a collapse and loss of function in related areas of the body, producing dysfunction or disease in a part of the body anatomically unconnected to the original source of the stress. This typically occurs first in the adrenal stress system and subsequently in susceptible aspects of the immune system. Having little or no reserves with which to continue to respond, the body becomes susceptible to assault from additional stressors. The result, at best, is usually a compromised immune system.

■ A Case History

For example, a couple of years ago I evaluated a pleasant and devoted woman who experienced a stroke while in her late seventies. Her pre-stroke life had been tumultuous, to say the least. Rest assured that she had paid her life dues prior to the stroke incident. Nonetheless, being the light-hearted individual she was, her inclination was to express an attitude of jovial optimism.

Even so, life recently confronted her with another extraordinary challenge. By nature, she is reticent to verbalize anything other than words of cheerfulness. Her disposition being what it is, she continued to display a good-humored, anti-victim attitude. However, it became quickly apparent that her capacity for processing this degree of life stress had been taxed. Although her resilient response to this most recent trauma required a Herculean effort, her internal stress response system had been overwhelmed.

Despite her ever-present smile and clever sense of humor, the effects of the trauma were more than she could process internally. Within days of the event, she began to scratch uncontrollably at multiple lesion sites that had begun to appear on her skin from head to toe. Being intimately familiar with her personal dynamics, it was a relatively easy task to determine the source of her problem.

This was the ultimate confrontation between psyche and soma. Over the years, her capacity for managing the effects of external assaults grew like the muscles of a world-class athlete. However, after a lifetime of actively processing life's little lemons into lemonade, her pitcher was full.

She grew up in an era of conflict and gripping world chaos. She was predisposed to making the most of everything. Appropriately, her ability to adapt became remarkable. However, one of her adaptive mechanisms included internalizing her natural responses to stressful situations. She was definitely not one to complain, let alone express negative feelings or emotions regarding her experiences. In fact, verbal communication was discouraged in the environment of her early maturity. With no outlet other than her adaptive capacity, she learned to mediate her encounters. But this time she stumbled upon one stress too many.

The price she paid was an unconscious and uncontrollable expression of the taxed psyche through the skin of her soma. Treating the symptoms proved fruitless, despite the well-intentioned efforts of her friends, family and physicians. However, the causal mechanism of her discomfort was quickly isolated and treated. Because of her highly developed ability to compensate for repeated exposure to stress, the actual mechanism allowing for the expression of symptoms was multifaceted. While it ultimately involved the immune system, elimination systems, and stress-response systems, it progressed due to nutrient deficiencies, compromised function, and loss of ability to compensate. Employing an aggressive combination of therapeutic nutrients, acupuncture, and relaxation techniques, the symptoms have since resolved, and she has regained her penchant for managing external influences through the use of her very highly developed stress response system.

However, her sole instrument for managing responses was so highly developed that it could easily have been misinterpreted as part of her personal dynamic, rather than as a sophisticated compensation mechanism. Even so, once the cause of her symptoms had been identified, a return to normal function was complete and swift. Frequently, these symptoms are so vague in their expression that they elude the sensitivity of traditional laboratory analysis until they are permanently fixed in the form of a recogniz-able disease.

■ Chronic Tonic

Meanwhile, the model upon which this overall approach to wellness is based is that of realm integration. Consider the following representation of a common scenario involving subtle discrepancies that accumulate in the relationship among the realms. Imagine a chronic exposure to one simple ingredient that is what it isn't: the habit of substance abuse, specifically alcohol. There is a body of evidence suggesting that in some forms and quantities, alcohol (particularly red wine) may be therapeutic. However, as we well know, in excess, it is considered a deadly toxin with extensive social, moral and physical complications. In many cases, by the time the abuse is identified, it is treated as alcohol abuse, instead of what actually shaped the abusive patterns that led to the symptoms being treated.

The following scenario is a common example of how this might occur. Imagine a fifty-year-old male in a high-stress job and an unhappy marriage who is forty pounds overweight. He is also sedentary, smokes two packs of cigarettes a day, and drinks a bottle of wine with his 8 p.m. high-fat meal. He suffers a heart attack and survives. He decides to quit his job (more stress), divorce his wife (avoidance stress), and initiates three hours of daily high-energy exercise stress. At the same time, he quits smoking and goes on a liquid protein diet (stress, stress and more stress). Ostensibly, his choices are good choices, but they are inappropriate to his circumstances. They are so extreme in nature that he will more than likely fall prey to some other unrelated pattern of behavior, leading to additional imbalances. Remember the caveat, "When you hear hoof beats, look for horses." All too frequently, the obvious is overlooked.

■ The Discovery of Insulin

The discovery of insulin as "a cure" for diabetes represents just such a phe-nomenon. The actual "scientific basis" upon which this belief is established is built upon the observations of researchers. They found that they were able to reproduce the high blood sugar symptoms of diabetes by damaging the pancreas of healthy animals. The conclusion is that the cause of diabetes is a deficiency in the production of insulin by the pancreas. Subsequently, it was found that the brain also produces insulin. So what else haven't we discovered yet that may be associated with the cause of an established disease? Is it possible that long-term abuse of a substance, such as white sugar, might result in actual diagnosable diseases, such as diabetes or attention deficit disorders, but not necessarily for the reasons we originally thought?

■ No Intrinsic Good or Bad

There are, of course, numerous examples of chronic imbalances producing symptoms that originate in all of the realms. Money can be a valuable tool used for many worthwhile endeavors. It can also be a curse. Exercise can be a productive element of a healthy lifestyle, but it also can be a stressful and harmful addiction. Food can be a medicine, or it can be abused to the extent that it becomes the source of innumerable health problems. Every drug of proven worth can itself produce a disease. Similarly, religion can be a source of inspiration and productive works, but when taken to the extreme, it can serve as the basis for fanatical behavior and extreme devastation. We begin to realize that there is no intrinsic good or bad, but simply where we stand in relationship to what we experience. Truth is where we find it, but at best, it is always only a partial bias.

Nowhere is this concept better illustrated than in the fable of the farmer whose wife left him shortly after the birth of their first son. His friends and neighbors proclaimed, "Oh what a terrible thing." But the farmer was left with a son who grew to be strong and healthy, someone to toil in fields and tend to his business. "Oh what a fine son, and how fortunate you are to have someone to assist in managing your business," the neighbors said. One day while riding, the son fell from his horse and broke his leg. What a terrible event. Two days later, representatives of the militia came to enlist the son as part of their warring army. Unfortunately, he was unable to go due to his disability. As you can imagine, the story, not unlike life itself, goes on and on. Experienced individually, these events present the opportunity to grieve or rejoice. We, too, are faced with the choice of clinging to grief as victims, or accepting it as an opportunity and a challenge through which we become more influential in managing our own lives.

■ Choosing How to Manage Our Experience

Seeking balance inevitably involves choosing how to manage experiences. This process depends to a large extent upon the nature of the concerns and the options one is willing to consider. The awareness with which alternatives are pursued dictates the context within which the alternatives chosen are received. Fate, destiny, and serendipity are all good words to describe the intangible process of evolution resulting from a sincere desire to improve existence. So, too, words can be chosen in the initial attempt of taking responsibility for interactions with the seen and unseen realms. This can further enhance active participation. Self-actualization can be initiated through simple attitudes, such as faith, conviction, intention, and affirmation.

The stress of life contains the seeds of spontaneity that produce the wonder of a new world. The awe inherent in the nature of existence can provide the motivation to greet each day expectantly, despite the possibility of dissatisfaction, despair, failure, and frustration. It is this unknown quality, this intangible possibility that sustains the hope and the belief that tomorrow can be better. And it can. But to exert some conscious influence over the outcome of tomorrow, awareness of the moment in which we now exist must be carried forth. Part of that awareness requires a cursory understanding of the mechanisms that regulate destiny. Another part requires a familiarity with the owner's manual and an understanding of how to operate the controls. As always, recognition of the fact that in each moment we affect and are affected by everything is obligatory.

■ Functional Diseases

Perceived as a whole, life seeks its own balance. The invitation to participate by the choice of our thoughts, words and actions is ever-present. Regardless, the beat goes on. Everything is what it isn't, depending upon the perspective from which it is observed. Further examining the possibilities for broadening an understanding of this paradox, the extent of its occurrence becomes obvious. Inquiry into every aspect of life produces the recognition of well-being as a dynamic interaction of cause and effect. Ideally, this interaction results in the homeostatic equilibrium of a productive and pleasurable outcome.

Events take place within our own bodies based upon what we are attracted to, what makes us feel good, and what we desire, with little or no consideration of the personal and public ramifications. Socially disruptive behavior and permissive interpretation of moral blueprints lead to chaos and corruption within our society. These then can be viewed as functional diseases of society. Too much or too little of anything demands a response. By virtue of the dynamic interdependence of the realms, every attempt will be made to restore equilibrium.

If too much sugar is eaten, too much insulin is produced. Short-term repetition of this behavior produces a multitude of symptoms. Frequently, these symptoms are ignored or misinterpreted, even as they result in the subclinical imbalance I discussed earlier, known as functional hypoadrenia. It is even possible for conventional medical belief systems to prevent a functional disorder from ever being correctly identified. They may never be associated with the underlying imbalance if they are not recognized or considered to exist. Remember, nothing exists until we observe it, even though the reality of its potential exists all the time.

■ Early Warning Systems

Functional hypoadrenia merely represents an early warning system. The stressors may be biochemical imbalances, emotional stress, financial stress, relationship stress, or almost any repetitive exposure to tension or anxiety-producing stimulation that can be imagined. The symptoms may include a wide variety of incessant related indicators. These can include weight gain, low energy, fatigue, sugar cravings, headaches, frequent colds and infections, elevated blood pressure and blood sugar, etc.

When the body's ability to manage the collective effects of these perceived stresses becomes overwhelmed, it begins pulling resources from other systems determined to be less important at the time. By the time the body runs out of options for managing the effects of the stress, there has been ample opportunity to treat one of the wide variety of symptoms as the problem. It is at this point that stress has the greatest possibility of becoming distress. However, a simple analysis of some basic functions reflected in the biological fluids quickly allows an early recognition of the symptoms as the body's cry for help in managing the assault.

In the case of attention deficit hyperactivity disorders, an early opportunity exists to identify the sources of the stress. Long before prescription drugs are recommended for the symptoms of ADD or ADHD several other possibilities must be explored. Hoof beats and horses must be examined from the start. Evaluating the nutritional status of the patient is fundamental to moving on to more exotic considerations. Environmental stresses, psychological profiles, and behavior should all be considered before the last resort efforts of managing symptoms with aggressive medications. Once identified, these alternative possibilities can be eliminated, minimized, or managed. Meanwhile, the objective of restoring proper function can be achieved by supporting the struggling system with appropriate raw materials, such as digestive enzymes, trace minerals, antioxidants, or specific system support. But in order for these possibilities to be included they must first be acknowledged. Nonetheless, we would be negligent to proceed any further without first seeking prerequisite advice from someone we presume to know—our doctor!

■ CHAPTER NINE ■
Ask Your Doctor

"Formerly, when religion was strong and science weak, men mistook magic for medicine; now, when science is strong and religion weak, men mistake medicine for magic."

—Thomas Szasz, The Second Sin (1973) "Science and Scientism"

■ Description of Prescription

The word "prescription"—abbreviated as "Rx"—has some interesting associations when applied to the virtual realm. As in medicine, a prescription can be a cure, remedy, or solution recommended to correct a disorder, imbalance, or problem. It can take the form of advice or information, which in the virtual realm is referred to as wisdom. Finally, a prescription is semantically related to a precept or guideline. This meaning can be extended to include a guiding rule or a set of activities undertaken as part of one's daily discipline. A virtual Rx then consists of remedies, wisdom, and recommended activities for those taking up a journey in the virtual realm. On the other hand, in today's society, the concept of a prescription has been repackaged to represent the promise of resolution in a pill, a procedure, a therapy, a diet, a piece of equipment, or involvement with a particular belief system, exercise routine, or investment group. As with any recommendation, prescriptions provoke some additional questions as to their efficacy, necessity, and side-effects.

Many people may have questions for their doctors about tests, surgery, therapy, recovery, drug treatment, risk factors, lifestyle changes, and other procedures. Few ever get to ask these questions, let alone get answers to them. There is much finger-pointing as to why. I state this here not to criticize doctors, but merely to demonstrate a point that is best illustrated by the following commentary.

On television, the drug companies make it sound as if you could talk to your doctor anytime you want to about anything. In all probability, these are disclaimers devised by their legal departments. The reality is that, aside from not having time to answer the suggested questions, most doctors don't really know the answers. Of course, many of them know what they've been told to say in response to questions about certain medications, but I'm talking here about really knowing. Nearly all doctors can respond adequately to questions concerning routine procedures with which they are experienced, but most doctors are far too inundated to have time to sort out the facts about procedures they have not used before with their patients.

Now facts, not unlike opinions, are not necessarily good or bad. They are usually just representative of a historical occurrence that can be used statistically to suggest any version of the truth to which one might subscribe. Sometimes, they can just be ignored altogether in lieu of conditioned response patterns to which the individual doctor has adapted. To demonstrate the commonness of these widespread perceptions, consider the impact of the following historical and statistical data.

■ Historical Facts

America was first in overall citizen health in 1900. By the beginning of World War II in 1941, we dropped to fifty-fourth. We rose back to number one before the war ended. Why? Primarily, because of food rationing and a return to home gardening and the development of the whole food store. Since that time, we have become world leaders in the technological manufacturing of artificial and preserved foods. We have also developed some of the most advanced medical institutions in the world to deal with the symptomatic results of these advancements. Meanwhile, our health status has continued to plummet to our current ranking as 100th in overall citizen health.

■ W.H.O. Study

Several years ago, a study done by the World Health Organization ranked thirty-three of the top industrialized nations on the planet in various categories of health. Considering our self-proclaimed role as the most advanced technological society in the world, and our arrogant aversion to researching alternatives, the results are most enlightening.

Out of the thirty-three nations evaluated, we ranked seventeenth in longevity. Sixteen other nations have populations who routinely live longer than the residents of the United States. Some of these include France, Italy, Portugal, and Japan. We were ranked twenty-third in the first year survivability of newborns. Twenty-two nations are documented to have a better chance of their babies surviving the first year of life than those born to residents of our high-tech medical society. Out of the thirty-three nations surveyed, we ranked last in the area of birth defects. Thirty-two nations have a lower birth defect rate than we do.

One of the most obvious contributing causes is that of our depleted nutritional resources in the food supply. Remember, if it's not in the soil, it can't be in the food. If it's not in the food, it's not in the diet. If it's not in the diet, it's not in the body. These facts alone should give us pause to reconsider our fundamental approach to the related statistics of degenerative disease and diet.

■ Higher Animal Standards

In fact, our animals are raised with a higher standard of basic health and nutrition than that available to our human offspring in the U.S. This is evidenced by the disparity in the rates of birth defects between humans and cattle. The current rate of human birth defects is one in 5,000. The rate of defects in the cattle industry is one in 500,000, or 100 times less than that experienced in the human population. In contrast, a cursory assessment of the nutritional resources available to human progeny and their counterparts in the animal kingdom discloses some rather disconcerting facts.

■ Questionable Human Standards

Of all the commercial infant food formulas available on the grocery store shelves, none currently has more than twelve minerals available as a constituent of the basic ingredients. Science Diet dog food has no less than forty. Lab rats are fed rabbit pellets with at least twenty-eight minerals. Mere coincidence, or do these facts suggest a healthier population of animals than infant humans?

Of course, the most obvious symptoms of childhood illnesses are written off as normal and routine. This is where sickness is considered to be an expected feature of the maturing process. For some reason, we assume this to be sensible. Is attempting to eliminate or minimize the causal factors unrealistic? Perhaps a notion as undemanding as "nutrients in and waste product out" is too simplistic for our sophisticated technological palate.

■ Prenatal Insanity

Meanwhile, the feeble attempts at prenatal nutrition contribute to the statistics. Political efforts to justify this behavior are based upon the partial truths of bogus studies performed by organizations with vested interests and ulterior motives. This is compounded by efforts to placate a population laden with functional learning disabilities by suggesting that pharmaceutical intervention presents the most viable alternative to managing these ravaging disorders. Rather than explore the possible relationship between normal function and adequate nutrition, we have opted for medicinal marvels to suppress the symptoms. All parties seem to be appeased by the passing of legislation that makes evaluation of the disorder available after the disorder is expressed as a symptom complex. This, then, is fully consecrated in the form of its own diagnosis code.

While the concept of supplementing the diets of developing children appears to be less absurd than escalated nutritional intervention three to six months prenatal, it is still far from a commonplace practice. Perhaps it is considered a fanatical obsession that would lead one to request some nutritional support in addition to the "prescription-only" formulas advocated by medical obstetricians, which typically contain all of four minerals essential to the normal biochemical environment in which the developing fetus will be expected to thrive.

■ Common Sense Dictates

Common sense would dictate that if in the first two weeks of life the nervous system (including the brainstem and the spinal cord) is the first structure to emerge and develop, it must have the essential elements available to do so with any degree of reliability. It seems obvious that the integrity of the developing system is dictated by the quality of the raw materials with which it is supplied. It seems equally apparent that the resulting system will most likely exert a high degree of control over what emerges as a consequence. This scenario alone would authenticate preconception nutritional support, as well as ongoing supplementation as the human embryo evolves.

It is not difficult to imagine how wide varieties of imbalance emerge as normal variants in a biochemical environment gone berserk. Further clouding the waters of common sense are the distorted perceptions of the balanced lifestyle required to support and encourage long-term wellness. Modern approaches to the models of health, diet, exercise, and nutrition, have done little more than confuse the issue.

The staggering levels of infertility and birth defects alone should lead us to examine the authenticity of society's opinions about what constitutes a healthy lifestyle. Is it actually realistic to assume that the high levels of birth defects, infertility, and miscarriage are chance happenings? Perhaps the innate wisdom of the body recognizes circumstances incompatible with life and communicates via an extreme response in the form of defect, miscarriage, or simply not allowing the process to be initiated? Are the myths of the predisposition for middle-aged birthing difficulties in our culture merely affirmation by an intelligence that recognizes a deprived biochemical environment in which it refuses to allow life to be conceived?

Yet, given these facts and observations, the commercial advertisement of medications as a way out suggests that we merely need to consult our doctor to see if a particular chemical is appropriate for our symptoms. In light of the probability that the body can actually think and manufacture its own solutions, this proposal becomes even more impractical.

■ Molecules and Receptors

Recall our previous brief discussion of molecules and receptors. Given that some form of innate intelligence orchestrates the millions of interactions occurring on a cellular level, we must assume that the body is aware of what's happening to it at any given point in time. Further, it is more likely than not that this awareness takes place at the level of the cellular receptor sites, as well as in the brain. Therefore, consider the following hypothetical application of these facts as an explanation for reactions that occur as the result of long-term use of pharmaceuticals.

The external introduction of a therapeutic chemical replaces the normal secretions of the body at the level of the receptors. Before going any further, a number of questions and concerns arise. First and foremost is the question, "Why isn't the body producing the substance?" Is the responsible structure damaged or impaired? Are the necessary raw materials absent or deficient? Nonetheless, a decision has been made to intervene with a man-made version of the lacking secretion. Several consequences (reactions to this action) begin to occur. Since what is known is all that is known about these preparations and the secretions they are designed to replace, what is not known is also not known. In all probability, this simple fact accounts for most, if not all, of the side effects of any man-made substitute.

■ A Reaction to Action

With the introduction of any foreign substance into the body, a series of known and unknown reactions begin to occur. The known reactions provide for the symptom relief of popular medications designed to resolve acid reflux, arthritis, fatigue, bloating, headaches, intestinal dysfunction, etc. The unknown reactions account for the side effects, as well as the long-term consequences of interrupting normal cellular exchanges.

When a receptor in the body is awaiting a particular communication and doesn't receive it, compensation begins to occur. When a partial message is delivered in the form of a pharmaceutical preparation, the receptor must act on the incomplete information. If this is the only information received over a long period of time, the receptor must adapt to this level of response. This causes adaptation to occur in all of the systems with which the receptor is designed to correspond. This leaves the body susceptible to the development of seemingly unrelated symptom complexes that might ultimately evolve into diagnosable diseases themselves. Long-term suppression of normal cellular communications has well-documented effects. These include alterations in the normal function of blood vessels, skin, brain, and fat cells, as well as progression into diagnosable diseases, such as diabetes, osteoporosis, ulcers, elevated cholesterol, internal bleeding, and immune suppression.

■ Practical Application

To illustrate a more practical application of this accumulated data, consider the conventional overview of a common diagnosable disease involving the thyroid gland. There are six commonly accepted symptoms of hypothyroidism. They include weight gain, dry skin and hair, hoarse voice, fatigue, cold intolerance and puffy facial features. So, you go to your doctor with one or more of these symptoms and some preconceived ideas about what is happening to you. At this point you have no formal diagnosis but you do have some thoughts about how you'd like to proceed and you just want to talk. But that's probably not going to happen, because your doctor has some ideas of his or her own, based upon the information and experience to which he or she has been exposed.

■ What Your Doctor Knows

It goes something like this: More than 10 million Americans have been diagnosed with thyroid disease, and another 13 million people are estimated to have undiagnosed thyroid problems. Frequently misunderstood, and too often overlooked or misdiagnosed, thyroid disease affects almost every aspect of health. So understanding more about the thyroid, and the symptoms that occur when something goes wrong with this small gland, can help to protect or regain good health. Sounds good so far! It's a concern that is widespread, can affect your overall health, and is obviously important.

A February 2000 research study at the University of Colorado Health Sciences Center, which was published in the *Archives of Internal Medicine*, found the estimated number of people with undiagnosed thyroid disease might be as high as 10 percent—*double* what was previously thought. This may mean that 13 million Americans are currently undiagnosed. Women are at the greatest risk of developing thyroid problems (seven times more often than men). A woman faces as high as a one in five chance of developing thyroid problems during her lifetime, a risk that increases with age, and for those with a family history of thyroid problems. It sounds as if we're learning something valuable here, so let's look a bit further.

■ Where Is the Thyroid and What Does It Do?

Your thyroid is a small bowtie or butterfly-shaped gland located in your neck, wrapped around the windpipe, behind and below the Adam's apple area. The thyroid produces several hormones, of which two are key: tri-iodothyronine (T3) and thyroxine (T4). These hormones help oxygen get into cells, and make your thyroid the master gland of metabolism.

The thyroid has the only cells in the body capable of absorbing iodine. The thyroid takes in iodine obtained through food, iodized salt, or supplements, and combines it with the amino acid tyrosine. The thyroid then converts the iodine/tyrosine into the hormones T3 and T4. The "3" and the "4" refer to the number of iodine molecules in each thyroid hormone molecule.

When your thyroid is in good condition, 80 percent of the hormones produced by your thyroid will be T4, and 20 percent T3. T3 is considered the biologically more active hormone—the one that actually functions at the cellular level—and is also considered several times stronger than T4. Once released by the thyroid, the T3 and T4 travel through the bloodstream. The purpose is to help cells convert oxygen and calories into energy.

As mentioned, the thyroid produces some T3. But the rest of the T3 needed by the body is actually formed from the mostly inactive T4 by a process sometimes referred to as "T4 to T3 conversion." This conversion of T4 to T3 can take place in some organs other than the thyroid, such as the hypothalamus, a part of your brain.

The thyroid is part of a huge feedback process. The hypothalamus in the brain releases thyrotropin-releasing hormone (TRH). The release of TRH tells the pituitary gland to release thyroid stimulating hormone (TSH). This TSH circulating in your bloodstream is what tells the thyroid to make thyroid hormones and release them into your bloodstream.

■ The Whole Truth?

This information is fascinating and true, but it isn't necessarily the whole truth. Whether intentional or not, this little story, convincing as it sounds, provides just enough pseudo-information to be dangerous. Some information extracted partially from historical data and partly from speculation, is combined with some truth to support the statistical and historical data presented. And there you have it: a belief system complete with recommendations for resolving a problem that may not even exist. Nonetheless, this presents quite a convincing story.

■ Contrived Presentations

Meanwhile, this is a typical and common presentation of information in response to the issues of physical and biochemical health. Taken at face value, it has little, if any, educational significance. It does provoke concern and point us in the direction of a traditional healthcare professional trained to assist in managing this problem. The potential problem here is that the people who perform the research, develop the data, and produce the products also provide the training.

Granted, the story sounds informative, cohesive, and convincing, but in the final analysis, it is still a story. It is associated with some products for managing the symptoms. These products are sold through local distributors at an inflated cost. Hmmm, sounds sort of like the world's biggest multilevel marketing company. But that couldn't be. After all, they would never deliberately deceive us for a profit, would they? Nah, I'm sure they have nothing but our best interest at heart. On balance, they did tell us how it works, and they did tell us who's at risk and what causes it. Why they even made recommendations regarding who to see and what to do about it.

■ Other Realities

To be fair, the other camp has assembled another reality for your consideration. Taking this same information and looking at it in a different way produces quite a different version of truth. It is a story about the relationship of historical and statistical data linked to some basic physiology. Assuming their motives to be somewhat similar, the story goes something like this: An overactive (hyperthyroidism) or underactive (hypothyroidism) thyroid can result in increased allergies, skin problems, fatigue, nervousness, gastrointestinal problems, sleeping too much or too little, gaining or losing weight, swelling, and various types of pain.

Of these two possible imbalances, hypothyroidism is the most common. Doctors are aware of the six basic symptoms associated with hypothyroidism.

But these symptoms are minor compared to the effects thyroid deficiency can have on the body, since every cell in the body needs thyroid hormone. You may experience any number of the "text book" symptoms, or none at all. Many people whose blood results are "normal" have debilitating symptoms of hypothyroidism and no hope of any help from the medical profession. Yet, if left untreated, you put yourself at risk for diabetes, high blood pressure, emphysema, arthritis, depression, migraines, and carpal tunnel syndrome.

Foods that depress thyroid activity include broccoli, cabbage, Brussels sprouts, cauliflower, kale, spinach, turnips, soybeans, and mustard greens. These foods should be included in the diet for hyperthyroid conditions and avoided for hypothyroid conditions. Also consider the following:

■ Avoid refined foods, sugar, dairy products, wheat, caffeine, and alcohol.
■ Essential fatty acids are anti-inflammatory and necessary for hormone production.
■ Take 1,000 to 1,500 mg flaxseed oil three times per day.
■ Calcium (1,000 mg per day) and magnesium (200 to 600 mg per day) help many metabolic processes function correctly.

■ Informative Propaganda

Now, before I go any further, let me stop here for just a moment and remind you of a caveat that can help to sort things out at this point in any story: When all you have is a hammer, everything looks like a nail. Typically, when these types of stories are constructed, regardless of their intention, they are associated with a particular product or service with which the individual presenting the story is associated by experience, by choice, or by both. Once again, this is not necessarily a bad thing, but it should definitely give one pause to acquire additional information surrounding the data presented and the recommendations being made.

For us to subscribe to a particular approach, it would be helpful to have further information about how recommendations relate to the cause of the symptoms. Of course, there is potential benefit to these suggested approaches, just as there is potential benefit to the nutritional recommendations, awareness of risk factors, and all of the other approaches with demonstrated advantages in isolated groups of cases. But, how do we decide which is most appropriate?

■ Hidden Meaning of Normal Tests

A more accurate appraisal of causal factors can be implemented when we use a more expansive model of assessment. By this, I mean looking beyond the symptoms, considering the whole person dynamics, and even looking at conventional test results in a different way. It is not unusual to be able to see a pattern of underlying imbalance demonstrated in an otherwise normal set of lab findings. The test is interpreted as normal because all of the values summarized in the test results are "within normal limits." Rarely are these tests looked at from the perspective of high and low normal values. All too frequently, an obvious configuration is overlooked because of the way something is looked at. Just because a specific test designed to demonstrate the existence of a disease comes back negative doesn't necessarily mean that a progression involving the suspected system is not in the process of developing.

As well, it may be helpful to investigate the symptoms through a different set of eyes. Some of the less conventional approaches to testing can also provide invaluable insight when considering symptoms that are low-grade, chronic, and unresolved. There are innumerable tests available for evaluating specific aspects of urine, blood, and saliva. Many other tests can be performed with simple tools, such as a blood pressure cuff and a thermometer. Several of these tests can assist in determining subclinical imbalances in isolated systems of the body, while suggesting simple, effective, and inexpensive solutions. Still others can elicit a DNA profile through an inner cheek swab that provides detailed information about function and genetic tendencies.

■ Differing Opinions

When reviewing different options for managing a group of symptoms resembling a disorder potentially involving something like the thyroid gland, other obvious issues inevitably present themselves. One is the somewhat confusing and conflicting nature of recommendations concerning nutritional support. Another is the tendency to ascribe a group of symptoms to a dysfunction in a particular system based simply upon the presence of the symptoms. It is valuable to remember that nothing experienced occurs in a vacuum. When considering the source of a group of symptoms, it is helpful to consider the tangible and the less tangible relationships in which the suspected system participates. For example, when dealing with the thyroid, there are some other possibilities to be taken into account. Two of these may not be directly reflected in the conventional assessments of the thyroid gland, but may actually involve the thyroid.

Since the thyroid gland has a specific relationship with the pituitary gland and the adrenal glands, involvement of one or the other as a primary source of imbalance may be misconstrued as a primary thyroid dysfunction. So, fundamentally, there are really three possibilities for functional thyroid involvement. The first is a primary dysfunction of the thyroid gland. The other two are imbalances in the pituitary or adrenals reflected as a thyroid involvement. Often these other two can be identified by the relationship of the levels in the other factors evaluated as part of a thyroid assessment. Specifically, this involves an expanded assessment of the blood and its components. Sometimes additional parameters must be tested to accurately isolate the source of the imbalance and associated dysfunction.

Since the thyroid gland maintains an active and intimate relationship with the adrenal and pituitary glands, an imbalance in either one can produce thyroid-like symptoms. The thyroid itself plays a major role in digestion and metabolism. The subjective indications for primary and secondary thyroid hypo-function can include morning headaches that wear off as the day progresses, resting muscle cramps, frequent infection, slow healing, chronic digestive problems, and excessive sleep requirements, to name a few.

Textbook hypothyroidism exists when symptoms and serum tests show elevated TSH (thyroid stimulating hormone from the pituitary telling the thyroid to work harder), low T4 (thyroxine produced by the thyroid and sent to the tissues), and low T3 (triiodothyronine converted from T4 to affect cellular metabolic processes). However, most of the time, hypothyroid symptoms and serum levels usually do not correlate very well. Several other peripheral chemistries, which are very helpful in confirming a suspicion, are too numerous to mention at this time. A brief general summary of an expanded approach is presented in the following illustration.

■ An Expanded Approach

Blood chemistries are the best way to determine which type of thyroid hypo-function to suspect. The following overview is presented as an example of how otherwise normal findings might be utilized in establishing the cause of related symptoms.

1. Primary thyroid hypo-function: T3 and T4 are low normal to decreased. Avoid foods in cabbage family, refined carbohydrates, dairy, fats and oils.
2. Thyroid hypo-function secondary to anterior pituitary hypo-function: TSH below 2.0, low to normal T3 and T4. Drink only pure water (no tap water or water containing chlorine or fluoride). Increase consumption of fresh fruits and vegetables. Eliminate refined, processed and fast foods. Eliminate hydrogenated fats or oils and all fried foods.
3. Thyroid hypo-function secondary to adrenal cortical hyper-function: TSH below 2.0, normal T3 and T4, potassium levels below 4.0, salivary cortisol normal in the morning and high all day. Drink plenty of water (no tap water or water containing chlorine or fluoride). Increase consumption of fresh fruits and vegetables. Eliminate refined, processed and fast foods. Eliminate hydrogenated fats or oils and all fried foods. Eliminate all alcoholic and caffeinated beverages.

■ What You Need to Know

When a thyroid dysfunction is being considered, the usual suspects must be evaluated, too! The best advice in any decision-making process regarding a course of action for any suspected malfunction is to remember that function needs to be thoroughly evaluated. Predictably, this process should begin with the known (when you hear hoof beats, look for horses) but it should not stop there. This also applies to alternative approaches, especially when selected merely for the sake of choosing an unconventional venue. Some people have had great success using only alternative medicine, while others must combine alternative and conventional.

Frequently, symptoms are so vague in their expression that they elude the sensitivity of traditional laboratory analysis until they are permanently fixed in the form of a recognizable disease. In the case of the potential thyroid involvement described above, it is just as likely that the thyroid-like symptoms are presenting themselves due to the functional hypoadrenia described earlier. This may be the early warning system suggesting that the body is compensating for a stress assault. The stresses can originate from any source of stimulation imaginable. Likewise, the symptoms can be portrayed in any form, or in any system of the body. What is seen is ultimately going to be determined by what is looked at and how it is interpreted.

■ Other Disorders Diagnosed as Diseases

Other examples of common disorders that are diagnosed as diseases and managed with medications might include elevated cholesterol, osteoporosis, obesity, depression, acid reflux, and heart disease. Even with these common, widespread disorders, there may be more than meets the eye. But the scenarios for evaluating and treating them are all very similar to those involving the thyroid.

Consider the common scourges of society that we're all reminded of through our exposure to the media, or our own family, friends, and co-workers. We know them by name. We even know the names of most of the common remedies for dealing with them. But is there any real hope available for eliminating them altogether? Your doctor might say, "Well now, just relax. Everything's going to be all right. Just take this pill and call me in the morning." Before we depart from the world of statistical and historical observation, there are a couple of more things we need to "ask our doctor." Let's start with something simple like cholesterol.

■ The Cholesterol Story

The latest research now shows some shocking facts about cholesterol. Elevated serum cholesterol is not a cause of heart attacks and strokes, as previously thought. Eating foods high in cholesterol is not a cause of elevated serum cholesterol, and therefore eating high cholesterol foods is not a cause of heart attacks and strokes. In fact, foods high in cholesterol and saturated fats (such as eggs, meat, fish, and poultry) will actually keep serum cholesterol down to normal levels. This is not to suggest, however, that high serum cholesterol is good. High serum cholesterol indicates the presence of a metabolic imbalance, but the high cholesterol component of that metabolic imbalance has no specific relationship to the risk of cardiovascular disease.

Elevated serum cholesterol is the result of the problem, not the cause of the problem. One of the most fundamental causes of atherosclerosis is not the presence of cholesterol, but the oxidation of cholesterol, which promotes the destruction of blood vessels by creating a chronic inflammatory response. This can lead to a series of events that may eventually lead to a heart attack or stroke. Fortunately, a comprehensive assessment, proper diet, and supplementation can go a long way toward identifying risk factors and resolving any accumulated damage due to these imbalances.

What this suggests is that the metabolic imbalance causing high serum cholesterol may increase the risk of cardiovascular disease. But if it does, it's not because of the elevated serum cholesterol per se, but because of a related elevation in triglycerides, homocysteine, C-reactive protein and low HDL cholesterol.

Now, the biochemistry gets a little intricate from this point on, so for the sake of brevity and reference, simply note that there are ten clinical indicators of cardiovascular disease risk and twenty-two causative factors of cardiovascular disease, according to the research available at the time of this writing. I mention this only to suggest that before we begin tampering with the effects of a system out of balance, we might be well advised to consider a broader perspective while educating ourselves as consumers.

■ Acid Reflux Disease

Another common example of the shell game of misinformation deals with the symptoms of a condition that is promoted as acid reflux disease. It is usually associated with overproduction of stomach acid. Actually, more times than not, it is a symptom created by too little stomach acid, not too much. Here's how it works. The stomach is basically a pressure organ. It performs its basic functions in response to pressure. Like the adrenals' indifferent response to the nature of stress, the stomach also does not care about the source of stimulation. It secretes its gastric juices in response to pressure. During a meal, pressure is created from ingested food and juices begin to flow.

Like everything else in the body, these juices must be replenished. They are created from raw materials extracted from the diet. If those raw materials are not present, they cannot be created. So when the next meal is eaten, there aren't enough juices to go around. The incompletely digested food putrefies, forms an acid and causes a burning sensation. Thus, in reality, reflux is caused by overeating, lack of raw materials to produce digestive juices, or from a condition called hiatus hernia, which causes abnormal external pressure on the stomach between meals, and is accompanied by the secretion of digestive acids into an empty stomach.

As for the other conditions I mentioned, as well as many more that I didn't, very similar scenarios exist. Once again, I have selectively organized a group of facts to support an opinion. There are as many, if not more, opinions available that could be constructed in complete opposition to what I have presented here. The point isn't who's right and who's wrong, because both are right and wrong. Remember, we only know what we know, and we don't know what we don't know. This fact contributes to how things are seen. Nevertheless, both camps regularly compile statistical and historical data in an effort to persuade new recruits to subscribe to a particular belief system. In so doing, the results are sometimes confusing and disconcerting, especially when a traditionally conservative and respected faction scrutinizes its own constituents. Take, for example, the following composite presented by an organization with a foot in both arenas.

■ Death by Medicine

"Death by Medicine" is an eye-opening paper published as a web exclusive in the March 2004 issue of *Life Extension*, a monthly magazine dedicated to "up-to-date coverage of the latest scientific and medical breakthroughs from around the world." As the grim title suggests, the paper explores the hazards of conventional medicine in the United States, analyzing and combining the complete published literature to date regarding injuries and deaths attributable to medicine. In their introduction, the authors note: "Never before have the complete statistics on the multiple causes of iatrogenesis been combined in one paper. Medical science amasses tens of thousands of papers annually—each one a tiny fragment of the whole picture .... Each specialty, each division of medicine, keeps its own records and data on morbidity and mortality like pieces of a puzzle.

"But the numbers and statistics were always hiding in plain sight. We have now completed the painstaking work of reviewing thousands and thousands of studies. Finally, putting the puzzle together, we came up with some disturbing answers." The "disturbing answers" the five researchers uncover are an indictment of the entire American medical system: "The total number of deaths caused by conventional medicine is an astounding 783,936 per year ... The number of people having in-hospital, adverse drug reactions (ADR) to prescribed medicine is 2.2 million.

"Richard Besser, of the CDC, in 1995, said the number of unnecessary antibiotics prescribed annually for viral infections was 20 million. Dr. Besser, in 2003, now refers to tens of millions of unnecessary antibiotics.

"The number of unnecessary medical and surgical procedures performed annually is 7.5 million ... The number of people exposed to unnecessary hospitalization annually is 8.9 million ... It is evident that the American medical system is the leading cause of death and injury in the United States."

They also project that the costs associated with deaths caused by medical interventions total approximately $282 billion per year, and estimate the costs for unnecessary hospitalization and medical procedures to total $16.4 million per year. The complete text of "Death by Medicine" can be found online at www.lef.org/magazine/mag2004. More than 150 references and an extensive appendix support the discussions and conclusions presented.

■ Look Again

Shocking? Yes! However, this information does appear to paint a rather unrealistic picture of conventional medicine. In so doing, it polarizes opinions and paints a noticeably bleak profile suggesting an "us versus them" scenario by presenting the information outside the context of the bigger picture. Subsequently, this otherwise valuable data blows the bad news out of proportion by alienating a viable faction of a necessary profession, and distorting a balanced opinion into a formal prejudice. Of course, we already recognize that everything works, and that includes traditional approaches to medical care.

Perhaps the only real discrepancy here is in the terminology, since the focus of conventional medicine is essentially disease management. Given this reality, and the fact that the hierarchy of established medicine attends to the vast majority of individuals seeking therapeutic attention, it seems a foregone conclusion that statistical data would reflect the associated performance ratios. Likewise, it seems that no similar analysis has been performed in the alternative community. Consequently, despite the flaws, failures, and shortcomings of the existing system, we lack the appropriate data to generalize such an opinion in looking at one aspect of a given segment of the healing arts.

In light of our caveats, it is important to keep an open mind when considering any approach to health care concerns. No appropriate decision can be made when based upon an opinion that contradicts or fails to consider the integrated dynamics of the realms. In review, it is always helpful to remember that:

- Anything can cause anything.
- For every action, there is a reaction.
- Everything works.
- There are no panaceas.
- When all you have is a hammer, everything looks like a nail.
- When you hear hoof beats, look for horses.
- Everything is what it isn't.

■ CHAPTER TEN ■
Doorway to Heaven

"Change your thoughts and you change your world."

—NORMAN VINCENT PEALE,
U.S. CLERGYMAN AND AUTHOR (1898–1993)

B y now, one thing should be very clear to you: Aside from the genetic and environmental influences of your early life, you are ultimately responsible for the choices you make. These choices, in turn, influence your personal experience of the realms.

The fundamental operating systems of reality, coupled with the innate characteristics of the physical and biochemical realms, lead to an inevitable challenge—how to use these tools to carve out an existence for yourself. While attempting to do this, a number of additional features come into play. Personal awareness, external stresses, belief systems, experience, purpose, passion, personality, preferences, and inborn traits all factor into the final results produced in your own life. The cumulative interplay of these essentials also dictates your contribution to the community consciousness of the human species.

Because there is a reaction for every action, you produce the details of your own personal experience. But you also play a part in developing the landscape in which all humans interact. The result is a universal dynamic, wherein we are all contributors and recipients. This platform provides an opportunity for each of us to impact the three realms of human experience.

■ Personal Contributions to Our Experience

Ultimately, the role you play in this interaction originates with the choices you make. These choices are embedded within the environment of your subjective experiences. The physical and biochemical realms then serve as the playing field for exchanges among the three realms. In a practical sense, this translates as the manner in which you experience outside stimuli and respond to it based upon your skill, familiarity, awareness, and development.

For instance, the choices you make regarding something like diet may be based upon habits adopted from your early years. If given little or no thought, these behaviors may have an impact on the length and quality of your life. They will influence the actions of everyone involved in providing you with the products you choose to include in your process. When you choose to purchase or use something, it has an impact on everyone involved in the process of producing that product and bringing it to market. If a particular food product is chosen on a regular basis, a positive economic impact is experienced by the owners of the land on which it is produced, as well as by the people who work the land, insure the workers, package the products, market them, sell them, distribute them, etc.

This is just one example of how we all affect and are affected by the choices that we make. These choices will also affect the environment in which they are produced and in which you live your life. As substances are consumed, the waste products must be managed. The way this waste is disposed of and the places it is deposited must be created, maintained, and changed in response to the nature and quantity of waste produced, while people must be educated and employed to monitor the costs, risks, and benefits of this whole process. Consequently, you play a vital role in the evolution of the underlying process of supply and demand.

■ Supply and Demand

In any society, the interaction of supply and demand is based upon behavior. In a best-case scenario, this information may encourage research based upon a statistical assessment of the dominant demands of any given population. This research can be funded by government and private sectors to determine the need, desire, cost effectiveness, and profitability, as well as to monitor trends, future demands, and alternatives for any given product. The availability of information pertaining to potential sources of supply ultimately allows a wider selection of options. Subsequently, you are able to exert more influence on suppliers for your behavior-related dollars by the demands you exhibit with your choices. More informed choices then become available.

But the marketplace can also manipulate these choices in terms of how the information gained in research is used to encourage behavior-related spending choices. In other words, once a trend has been recognized, identifying what caused people to respond to the product in the first place can be used to encourage people to purchase more of it. If it is a food product and taste is the most popular aspect of the product, any number of things can be manipulated to enhance the taste and encourage more buying.

For instance, numerous additives can be incorporated to stimulate cravings and even addictions to the food. Visual images of the food can be presented in such a way so as to make the food more desirable, or to make you believe that you will be more desirable if you eat it. This is true with any popular product and its related image. If you believe that somehow your life will be better by having, wearing, eating, living in, or driving something, then you can be assured that all of those things will be readily available in the marketplace for your consumption.

From the perspective of supply and demand, this entire scenario directly impacts your physical and biochemical environments. As the number of supply choices widens, there is a greater focus on the by-products created in the process. The net effect of consumer choices on things such as pollution, the economy, depletion of the soil, and degradation of the water supply produces a very real influence on the world we live in. They are a direct result of the choices we all make individually and collectively.

■ Overlooking the Forest

The last hundred years have produced miraculous discoveries and an ever-widening sphere of knowledge and information. However, it is easy to get lost wandering in this forest, never becoming aware of the trees. Because of the speed and volume of available information, we often fail to extract and incorporate the truly meaningful features of this resource. It's easy to become overwhelmed.

More often, the actual information produced is shrouded in a deluge of media hype. While designed to inform, it frequently confuses and misleads. All too often, a sound bite of truth extracted from a larger database of research is exaggerated, distorted, or disguised to create a false impression. This process is commonly referred to as advertising and marketing. Step back for a moment to examine this dynamic, and it's easy to see how this happens. Once aware of these tricks, it is easy to develop an effective approach for evaluating information and making more informed choices.

■ The Mechanisms of Choice

Much of what is chosen is based upon exposure and experience. It is also related to a basic fear of the unknown. The nature of this fear revolves around being separated from a source, located somewhere outside of yourself, that is responsible for nurturing and supporting you. The fear is that this separation will cause you to be deprived of the ongoing nurturing and support. This fear generates fear-based behavior that is rooted in attempts to re-establish this relationship so that you can be reinstated in the good graces of the provider. Right, wrong, or indifferent, this is often the basis for allegiance to organized religious belief systems.

A new study has backed up these findings, and provided some tentative explanations for this surprising phenomenon. Many people believe in a God, but don't go to church, pray or otherwise follow through much on that belief. This may "raise the specter of punishment after death without hope for salvation," wrote the researchers, Paul Wink and Julia Scott of Wellesley College in Wellesley, Mass., in a paper describing the findings. Fear of death "was particularly characteristic of individuals whose belief in a rewarding afterlife was not matched by their other religious beliefs and practices." They're afraid of punishment in the afterlife, such as going to hell.

The other aspect of this fear is that it produces a vulnerability that is catered to by advertisers who appeal to basic desires, wants, and contrived needs. It is this fear that motivates you to seek the approval of others, attempt to control events, and associate yourself with external symbols of power. Both aspects of this fear create a predisposition to behave in anticipation of a response. Both produce a transitory effect that exists only as long as the object of reference is present in your life. This accounts for the tendency to acquire more credentials, power, possessions, and status. However, this generates yet another fear, that of loss. This fear increases with age and recognition that the nature of the material world is temporal.

As discussed earlier, experience leads to desire, and desire leads to intentions to either re-experience or avoid experiencing certain events. Intention then focuses attention, which increases the probability of an experience reoccurring. Information is manufactured in such a way that it is accepted as truth for one of two reasons. Either, you really want to believe it, or you're afraid not to believe it. In either event, the fear is well represented by the acronym described earlier: F.alse E.vidence A.ppearing R.eal.

This, then, is the underyling motivation that produces all experiences in all three realms. When the dynamics of a quantum lifestyle are more closely examined, this underlying dynamic can be consciously employed to directly affect experiences at a causal level. This means that you can learn to establish your reality by creating your thoughts through the application of practices that will assist you in developing the discipline of deliberate intention and focused attention.

■ The Power That Binds Us

The universal intelligence that orchestrates everything in existence is located in the virtual realm. But its effects are far-reaching. It coordinates the efforts that are imposed upon it into a biophysical dialogue through which communication in the material world occurs. It basically resembles a kind of cosmic putty that is constantly remodeling itself to produce the desires, wants, and needs impressed upon it by the intentions we submit. Its response is very similar to the squeaky wheel syndrome in that the most focused attention to intentions becomes the dominant tangible manifestation of this all-pervading and sustaining source. Every groundbreaking discovery and world-changing event got its start in the potential of the unseen realm. As the potential of each recurrent behavior is realized, the probability of it being repeated is enhanced. It is through this mechanism that the familiar aspects of life are experienced. While this can be good—and even helpful when it comes to making a long distance phone call, crossing an intersection, or even depositing money into a bank account, for example—there is a dark side, as well.

Once these methods have been studied and interpreted, the means by which they function can be identified and used for any intended purpose. Specifically, when patterns of behavior are analyzed, the demands of the marketplace can be tailored to tap unseen feelings. This is called market research analysis. Unfortunately, incorporating the analysis of trends with motivational tools based upon basic wants, desires and needs may artificially create a demand in the minds of consumers. The result is the transmission of partial truths embellished with a sense of urgency or subtle fear that panders to basic desires.

These transmissions are managed by a part of the brain called the reticular activating system (RAS). This network provides an alerting or arousal function. The cells in this structure are activated by novel sensory stimuli and remain highly active during states of arousal. Specific hormones are involved in regulating these activities. This system processes incoming information and contributes via the biochemical realm to the overall consistency of physical experiences.

However, unless vigilance is maintained, it is easy to unwittingly become the victim of external manipulation. This manipulation occurs through exposure to external stimulation designed to encourage specific thoughts or to produce specific actions. It also occurs as a result of the communal influences of others responding to these stimuli, otherwise known as herd consciousness. Have you ever noticed how everyone seems to be going to the same place at the same time? Listen closely as the volume of the next commercial indiscreetly goes up when you leave the room to raid the fridge. Watch intently as the same close out sales and limited time offers are presented on a regular basis.

■ The Attributes of Existence

One of the attributes of existence is that everything vibrates or resonates at its own particular frequency. These frequencies are unique to every component of each of the realms. Composite frequencies are the cumulative effect of everything that everyone is exposed to in each of the realms. The conscious mind is aware of less than one-tenth of one percent of the information that comes into the senses: that's sixteen bits out of 40 million per second! Consciousness acts like a sieve straining out the vast bulk of information received through the senses. As a result, hidden intelligence rooted in the virtual realm works more effectively through the subconscious mind, than it does through the conscious mind.

Everyone has an innate ability to fine-tune his or her own resonance to pick up information anywhere and anytime. It is not a question of learning how to resonate. Everyone already instinctively knows how to do this. It is more a question of learning how to consciously alter internal frequencies to match those of people and things with which interaction is desired. This opens up new pathways for communication and understanding.

Within everyone, there is a river of veiled intelligence. Beneath the noise and turbulence of our conscious minds lies a hidden realm of awareness whose existence may not even be realized. This river of potential flows all the time through our changing seasons of emotions, physiological conditions, and mental states. Most importantly, this river can be accessed at anytime. It provides us with a compilation of intuitions, hunches, and gut feelings, based upon desire, intention, attention, and motivation.

We experience the results of repetitive interaction with this creative source in the form of our life experiences. These experiences can be very healthy, productive, and encouraging. But learning to access the source of them intentionally means learning how to minimize exposure to counterproductive stimuli that might distract our attention and pollute the intended results.

This becomes particularly relevant when thinking about our routine exposure to newspapers, television, radio, books, magazines, and advertisements. All media is designed to communicate to the senses in the range of frequencies they are capable of perceiving. Once aware of this fact, the number of attempts to manipulate behavior through the five senses becomes amazing. While these external messages might appear to represent information, they also contain carefully constructed formats that help to inspire a predictable response. The more one is exposed to these messages, the more one is likely to respond the way marketers intended.

■ Extrasensory Communication

Each of our five senses is capable of receiving information that vibrates and resonates within a specific range of frequencies. You're accustomed to receiving information within the range of frequencies that each sense is capable of translating. Subsequently, you automatically assume that "That's all there is." Nothing could be further from the truth. This is evidenced by the fact that other frequency ranges have been identified, and instruments have been developed to interpret these communications. Infrared, microwaves, radio waves, X-rays, and gamma rays are but a few examples of this unseen world of everyday influences. Remember, you can only know what you know, and you don't know what you don't know. Will Rogers said this a different way: "We're all ignorant, just about different things."

Since all creation is manifest from energy, the smallest components of existence exist as pure energy. The density of an object is what governs how fast that energy can physically vibrate. Objects must vibrate within certain ranges of frequency for human senses to perceive them. A major factor that limits people from readily perceiving higher frequencies is that the frequency rate of vibration is outside the range of human perception. This contributes to a lack of faith and an inability to believe in something that cannot be perceived through the normal senses. The fact is that evidence of the existence of extrasensory communication bombards humanity each and every day. Even though something can't be directly perceived doesn't mean that it doesn't exist. For example, blowing on a dog whistle produces a very real sound for a dog that cannot be heard by the human ear. But the sound is real as perceived by a dog. Its range of perception is different than that of a human but this doesn't make the sound any less real.

■ Monitoring Your Exposure

The bulk of our conscious communication is delivered through the five senses. It is within these perceptible frequency ranges that all information compiled by mankind is consciously transmitted. Therefore, if desire is propagated by our attention to past experience, pleasure can be intentionally created and deliberately communicated through frequency ranges perceived by the senses. Everyone is basically seeking to attract pleasurable experiences and avoid painful ones. The available frequencies can be used to deliberately encourage pursuit of pleasurable experiences by virtue of the information and images transmitted along within them. If an intention is fine-tuned by attention, then whatever pleasurable frequencies are chosen for sensory exposure will likely dictate the vibrational frequency of the resulting experience. Consciously working to increase the rate of vibration will assist in developing the ability to perceive communications from within the virtual realm by increasing the vibrational sensitivity of our intentions.

Standing between what's been experienced and what is yet to be observed, it appears as though everything originates in and returns to the virtual realm. The virtual realm thus exerts a dramatic and powerful effect, communicating and responding through the biochemical conduit into physical experience. So, then, the virtual realm represents an opportunity for us to participate consciously in the creation of our own life experiences. It is ironic that so much time, money, and energy are spent attempting to quantify, regulate, control, and alter the effects experienced in the two tangible realms (physical and biochemical). Ultimately, however, we must recognize that the cause of these effects is mediated within the virtual realm itself.

■ What If?

Stop for a moment to reflect on the concerns that seem to plague us. Then, think about the enormous opportunity that conscious cooperation with the virtual realm could offer. What if simply readjusting our tuning frequencies could resolve all of the issues we perceive as problems? What if one could consciously engage the creative process to produce anything desired, anytime it was wanted? What if we are already doing this, but are simply unaware of it? What if we cultivated skills necessary to live life the opposite from the way we've been living it? What if, instead of struggling with issues of daily life and frantically enduring an unsatisfying existence, other choices were made?

With evidence mounting that life may just be about making choices, attention may have been focused on the wrong things for quite some time now. It may not be all about the genetics of birth, the environments people are raised in, or the stressful responses to inherently neutral external stimuli. It may not be about the external manifestation of symptoms arising in an individual's life that need to be conquered. It may simply be about monitoring responses and managing the decision-making process.

■ The Cure May Be in the Cause

The cure for all major diseases may not be in the next pill, or the next therapy. It may be in examining the reasons why these concerns are so abundant that we begin to explore potential causes, rather than "cures." The reasons people are unhappy, unfulfilled, depressed, anxious, or angry may not reside in chemical changes that occur as a natural part of the aging process. They may reside in the way things are looked at, the way change is responded to, or the way one thinks and has thought throughout the course of a lifetime.

Two Related Case Histories

I can recall two specific cases of this involving massive skin eruptions covering the entire body. In both instances the eruptions were evaluated conventionally and determined to be of unknown origin. Medications designed to assist in controlling the symptoms were prescribed. By the time I evaluated these cases, one had been unresolved for approximately eighteen months, and the other for two years. Both patients were males. One was in his late thirties and the other in his late forties.

Following the initial consultations, comprehensive surveys were completed. Nutritional assessment determined that both patients had extremely distorted profiles. Nutritional intervention was prescribed in conjunction with dietary proposals.

The thirty-eight-year-old male had suffered for almost two years with his condition. During the course of treatment, conversations with him revealed that prior to the onset of his "skin condition," he had become addicted to alcohol. This addiction had caused him to lose his job, his wife, and his child. Tormented by these losses, he spiraled deeper into his addiction. By the time he consulted with me, he had been assigned a total disability status. He was also covered head-to-toe with bandages and was taking twelve different medications daily. He had also lost almost fifty percent of his hair, due to his frequent scratching of the lesions.

Initially, his biochemical environment improved dramatically. But there was no obvious improvement in his external symptoms. As he became more comfortable sharing the intimate details of his prior life, he became more receptive to my suggestions of working with the feelings he was experiencing. Meanwhile, we continued to monitor and modify his biochemical environment.

Over the next three months, his skin condition improved by fifty percent. He was now able to interact socially without the bandages and was able to dispose of eight of the twelve medications. Over the next six months, his skin disorder was completely resolved, his hair all grew back, he started a new job, and he no longer indulged in alcohol. In the months that followed his recovery, he also was reunited with his family. This occurred in 1998, and to my knowledge, he remains healthy, active, and productive to this day.

The other gentleman had been suffering from his skin lesions for about eighteen months when I first met him. We engaged in a process similar to the one I described above. With treatment, his biochemical environment improved consistently over a period of six months, but there was no change in his skin condition. He was a wealthy and successful entrepreneur who traveled a lot for his business. He insisted that, other than the condition that plagued him physically, everything else in his life was perfect. Unfortunately, this turned out to be not quite true. During the course of numerous dialogues designed to address the other arenas of his life experience, he shared numerous events that concerned him. But he persisted in refusing to acknowledge any relationship between these circumstances and his skin disorder.

At my suggestion, he took some time off to attend a series of programs that offered him an opportunity to relax in completely stress-free, therapeutic environments. During the course of his participation in these programs, his condition resolved itself completely and remained that way for several days following a return to his normal lifestyle. Inevitably, his chronic skin condition gradually returned within weeks following his homecoming. Despite this fact, he refused to acknowledge any relationship between his everyday life and his symptoms. The last time I saw him, his skin condition had once again reemerged. We had a final discussion concerning the likely dynamic involved, and we talked about some realistic approaches to resolving his problem. As of this writing, however, I have not heard from him or seen him since that time.

■ Virtual Imbalances

One third of my patients demonstrate a similar phenomenon. For example, I recently participated in the care of an eleven-year-old female whose chief complaint was that of stomachaches. While the physical evaluation was essentially negative, her biochemistry was substantially distorted. Treatment demonstrated consistent biochemical improvements, however there was no apparent change in her stomachaches. Upon further inquiry, I discovered that she had been estranged from her birth father for quiet some time. Recently, communication had been reestablished, and the father had agreed to a trial reconciliation with the family.

In preparation for this reunion, she would have to withdraw from school and relocate to another state. With her having made all the necessary preparations, her classmates threw her a going-away party as a final gesture of farewell. Weeks later, the father reneged on his decision, and the child was faced with embarrassment, ridicule, frustration, contempt, disappointment, and a deep hurt over this change in plans. Unable to adequately express her deepest feelings, her concern was expressed as a stomachache. Once this cause was unmasked, her situation was resolved. She is now learning how to communicate and adapt, thus restoring balance from a virtual perspective, while we continue to treat the biochemical effects of this upset.

In two similar, but unrelated, cases, two female patients both expressed physical symptoms that were attributed to menopause. Yet there was no objective, physical evidence to support this proposal. With the physical diagnostics accounted for, a nutritional evaluation was performed. Both demonstrated severe imbalances that were subsequently addressed. While some of the superficial symptoms improved, the more severe concerns of depression, anxiety, insomnia, and fatigue persisted. Both had experienced recent weight gains, excessive cravings, and skin rashes in conjunction with their other symptoms. As their biochemistry improved, the core symptoms persisted. Pursuing a virtual prospect, it was disclosed that each had good reasons for their persistent symptoms. The male child of one of the women had just been convicted of murder and sentenced to life in prison.

The other's husband had left her, and she had no means of support, no skills, and no hope. Both currently continue to be monitored in my office, while receiving the appropriate supportive care to address causal imbalances rooted in the virtual realm. Remarkably, once the cause of the symptoms was identified, acknowledged, and addressed, both have reported losing weight, feeling more energy, having less cravings, sleeping better and feeling more confident and positive about their lives.

■ A Stroke Is Just a Stroke?

Finally, I'm reminded of a jovial young lady of age eighty-three who suffered a spontaneous stroke. Prior to this incident, she was vibrant and active, with a great sense of humor. Within weeks of recovering from the initial impact of this experience, she came to my office in her wheelchair. The stroke had compromised her physical mobility. One of the apparent secondary symptoms was an elevated blood pressure. With the normal acceptable range for blood pressure being 120/80, hers was roughly 190/110. However, she remained optimistic and energetic. She was anxious to engage every opportunity for recovery, despite the inconvenience of her impairment.

Her right arm and leg had been primarily affected, with loss of any ability to move or feel. Armed with little more than her great attitude and supportive family, we began an aggressive course of acupuncture, neuromuscular therapy, and nutritional intervention.

Within eight weeks of beginning her rehabilitation, she had achieved complete use of her right arm, with a seventy-five percent improvement in her right leg. Within the next four weeks, we were able to withdraw all medications, including those prescribed for her elevated blood pressure, which was now stable at 110/82. Within the next four weeks, she was able to participate in activities with the assistance of a walker. As of this writing, it has been two years since the initial incident. She remains stable, active and an enthusiastic inspiration to the members of her community and family. She is now capable of walking on her own, assisted by a walker. She uses the walker, not because of any residual symptoms from the stroke, but because of complications following a knee replacement. Searching for the cause of the stroke in this case was a relatively mute point. An attitude of gratitude and expectation propelled this buoyant person into aspects of the virtual that quickened a return to wholeness. There is a lesson here for all of us.

■ Two Other General Categories of Imbalance

There are two other general categories of imbalance that are equally prominent in my day-to-day clinical experience. The first involves a straightforward dynamic of causal factors originating within the realm in which the
symptoms express themselves. A common example is a physical injury
sustained in some sort of physical activity or accident. Another might be a
full-fledged biochemical imbalance, originating and expressing itself in the
biochemical realm. The simplest forms often involve some form of nutritional imbalance or deficiency. The hallmark of single realm–single cause
symptom complexes is that, once identified, they tend to resolve quickly
and completely.

The other category of imbalance is similar to those described earlier.
These involve the virtual realm as a point of causal origin. In these cases,
the causal factors often appear pretty straightforward, but remain resistant
to the obvious attempts to resolve them. Also, they often create dramatic
effects in one or both of the other two realms. These tend to be more difficult to identify and treat, since a significant degree of layering or masking
has already occurred.

■ A Final Word

There are also innumerable methods available for assessing and evaluating
each suspected cause. But since everything works, the most appropriate
tools must be selected to achieve a specific goal. Initially, this can be a little overwhelming, just because of the shear volume of available options.
Take, for example, the condensed version of the examination for becoming
credentialed in internal medicine. The review for this examination alone
consists of some 46,000 questions. When all of the specialties in conventional medicine that are designed to assist in diagnosing existing disease
processes are included, the pool of potentially relevant data becomes staggering. And that is just the result of information observed and accumulated
pertaining to the function of the physical body.

All of the descriptions, definitions and examples incorporated to this
point in the book have been included to provide information and perspective. Obviously, the various elements I chose to incorporate are not all-
inclusive. There are literally an infinite number of factual observations that

could be made to establish and justify an opinion as to how any of these three realms originated, developed, and function.

My purpose in presenting the selective facts associated with each of the realms is to create awareness, respect, and insight regarding the tangible aspects of our human experience. Both the physical and biochemical realms are directly observable as effects produced by an underlying creative intelligence. In contrast, the virtual realm is unobservable, except for the effects created in the other two realms.

The virtual realm is not only the most important of the three realms, but the source of all three. Meanwhile, despite the speculative and intangible nature of the virtual realm, many of its characteristics have been identified, interpreted and verified through the application of reproducible scientific investigation. When considering the related aspects of all three realms, the possibilities are literally infinite.

■ CHAPTER ELEVEN ■

Quantum Lifestyle Dynamics

"The second half of a man's life is made up of nothing but the habits he has acquired during the first half."

—FYODOR DOSTOEVSKY, RUSSIAN NOVELIST (1821–1881)

The goal is to develop a working model for behaviors that lead to a life of conscious co-creation and fulfillment. But first, a useful reality must be constructed based upon information that can produce predictable and reproducible results in our day-to-day lives.

In essence, any lifestyle discipline that includes self-assessment ensures personal growth, self-awareness, and spiritual security. In fact, spiritual security can be gauged by how someone feels most of the time. As the unknown becomes more familiar, the fear of the unknown dissipates. Such is the goal of all the age-old systems for achieving inner peace, personal growth, wisdom, contentment, and salvation. The notes in the songs may vary, but the melody is always the same. Ten steps to ... Seven keys of ...

Three ways to ... etc. Formulas for improving, enhancing, accelerating, and establishing are manufactured from the language into well-intentioned dialogs of support and encouragement. These countless prescriptions provide guidance, inspiration, and motivation.

But these words can only lead us to the experience. Even so, they are necessary to promote advancement toward the creative source from which they emerged. And so, I too, will use some of these words combined in a little different way to offer a distinctive view of the unseeable. Understand that these words have been selected to represent my personal impressions and perspective. They are not a system or a means to anything. Rather, they represent an instrument used to compose a symphony that resonates as a melody for sharing observations about the nature of a quantum lifestyle.

One only has to look as far as their own situation to recognize what isn't working for them. Oftentimes, this appears as a symptom in the form of a recurring situation or relationship. At times, it may be an unresolved feeling or chronic physical discomfort. Often, it simply appears as a deep sense of unrest and imbalance. Not really knowing what it is that's causing the disturbance, the first inclination is to grasp at the popular, easy, quick, and available solutions only to find that, along with a temporary change, another problem has been created.

Statistically, it is known that the highest percentage of failures is not because people don't want to have healthy, productive and prosperous lives. More times than not, it is because they don't know how to achieve such a life. Thus, it is the use of a flawed system, rather than the lack of motivation or commitment, that produces a less-than-desirable result. Discouragement and complacency are common by-products of the frustration experienced while attempting to achieve a desired result and continually failing to succeed.

These are usually symptoms, not terminal conditions, and ultimately result in a lack of motivation and commitment. The presence of symptoms in the absence of diagnosable disease suggests an imbalance. This imbalance is created by a repetitive sequence of events originating in the thoughts of the experiencer. This type of vicious cycle is self-perpetuating once it gains critical mass in one's life. However, the associated symptoms need not become a chronic lot in life.

■ Conditional Responses

Although you may have been conditioned to respond to certain types of external stresses in a particular way, you have the ability to alter the outcome by virtue of how you choose to respond to the situations, circumstances, or encounters interpreted as a source of stress.

Repeatedly allowing an external stimulus to dictate your response perpetuates the illusion of separation, in that you ascribe the source of your chosen response to the stimulus. Once you realize that touching a hot stove will burn you, you realize that the result of touching it again will produce the same experience. It is not the hot stove that burns you, but your decision to touch it. The illusion of separation is further perpetuated by our identification with the hot stove as the source of the burn, rather than with the decision-maker who chose to touch it.

■ Hidden Meaning of Behavior

Likewise, blaming falsely assigns responsibility to a person, object, or circumstances for your experience of the encounter based upon your subjective interpretation. Considered in this light, accidents become opportunities to look at things differently. And they should, particularly if they keep occurring as part of your life experience.

Taken to the extreme, chronic blaming may suggest that an unfulfilled need for attention, caring, cuddling, or nurturing is being fostered. This dynamic may work to satisfy needs and longings for everyone in support of the contrived relationship. By the same token, it may reinforce the thought patterns associated with one's own self-image, creating a terminal dysfunction of dependency and self-flagellation. This can prevent you from accessing any other life experience. This behavior may get you what you think you need, but not necessarily what you really want. Besides, it is a lot of work for very little return. What we're looking to achieve in deliberately constructing a process is the biggest return from the least investment. But as always, the choice is yours for the choosing. The concept of six degrees of separation suggests the mathematical probability that we are never more than five or six people away from any relationship we desire. I am suggesting that we are never more than one thought away from any experience we choose.

■ Three Things We Must Know

Therefore to alter your experience consciously and deliberately, you must know three things. Firstly, you must recognize where you are. Secondly, you must know where you want to be. And thirdly, you must know how to get from here to there.

Self-observation is at the core of any truly effective endeavor to shape productive and intentional changes in life. A loosely structured approach to self-examination follows a classical pattern of differential diagnosis, while providing a powerful basis for refocusing your efforts in the direction of correction. A variety of tools, in the form of caveats, guidelines, reminders, and suggestions, have been presented throughout this book. These represent prerequisite elements of a system that can be combined to create whatever you desire and help to keep you on track.

■ Acknowledge Where You Are

Recognizing that everything works, one quickly realizes that there are no panaceas. You can begin to construct a unique approach to experiencing the reality of your dreams by starting where you are with the "hoof beats" caveat. When you hear hoof beats, look for horses. In so doing, you accomplish the first step in the process of self-renovation. You acknowledge where you are. Given the facts of our discussion about the characteristics of thought and the nature of "now time," there really is no other place to start.

The symptoms will vary from person to person at this stage of our journey. And quite frankly, they really don't matter. They are just symptoms. But more importantly, they are self-generated guideposts to a solution. Remember that everything is what it isn't. The solution is always in the problem, and the symptoms can provide invaluable insight into where the imbalance exists and what possible remedies are available.

In the final analysis, it will always boil down to one simple concept anyway. The main problem is that you think something is wrong. However, for most of us, it is a difficult diagnosis to convert into a remedy at this point, so you must employ some strategic impetus to move in the desired direction. Remember, for every action, there is a reaction. Doing nothing produces more of the same. Just doing something for the sake of doing something will simply produce random and inconsistent results. This leads to either more confusion, or more of the same.

■ Specific Action Produces Specific Reactions

Using the three things you have to know as a foundation for creating a new experience, you must now begin to refine your efforts to accomplish your goal. Creating a system that works for you is critical to achieving and maintaining motivation and consistency. This does not require you to subscribe to a specific belief system or dogma, but only to align yourself with practices that produce predictable results and are consistent with your fundamental desires.

To produce results consistent with your desires, you must consistently apply the principles of manifestation in as conscious a manner as you are capable in any given moment. You can use the laws, guidelines, caveats, and reminders to construct a realistic program for successfully altering your course and restoring balance, while establishing a self-perpetuating foundational awareness. The more specific you are at each point along the way, the more specific your results will be, and the easier it will become to monitor progress and modify your approach.

Starting where you are will be as different for everyone as individual perceptions of reality. Despite the fact that everyone wants the same basic things (avoiding pain and experiencing pleasure), your plan for achieving these results will be different. What will be the same, however, is the fundamental mechanism for achieving it. Universal laws are called universal for a reason.

■ Anatomy of a Successful Experience

In attempting to achieve mastery over the circumstances of life, you are frequently encouraged to examine the lives of successful people. In reality, you can examine anyone's life to dissect out the key elements contributing to their present situation. The same laws produce what you interpret as success and failure. The basic operating system is infallible. It always generates predictably consistent results. So you are merely observing the application of principles that produced the results and concluding them to be good, bad, or indifferent. This observation is always made from where you are looking at it, and is rarely an accurate assessment of how someone else is experiencing it.

Words of Wisdom

- Expectation is 90 percent of manifestation.
- Words bring your expectations into your experience.
- The instructions you follow determine the reality you create.
- Your outcome is only as good as the system you employ.
- The best predictor of future behavior is past behavior.
- When you choose the behavior, you choose the consequences.
- You get what you give, so give what you want to receive.

The fact that you are where you are is because you are where you are. Given this as a starting point, you can begin to identify where you want to be and how to get there. In addition, you can begin to explore the three major influences to which everyone is susceptible. Again, these include genetics, environment, and stress. Although these three influences are the same for everyone, your experience of the influences will be different. Why? Because everything is what it isn't.

So now you have what you must know, and you know what you have, but the next step is to know what you must have. There are three key components or characteristics associated with all deliberate creations. First, you must have the desire or motivation to create something. Next, you must have a system for creating it. And lastly, you must have a commitment to creating it. While a system failure is the number one reason for creating something other than what you imagined, the second most common reason for failing to alter an outcome is a lack of consistency or commitment to a system that works. And since everything works, you are really experiencing the result of a principle of fabrication that states, "You get what you give." In other words, when you give your attention to what you want, it sets in motion a chain of unseen mechanisms for producing it.

Employing the suggestion of changing the way you look at things, this principle suggests a fundamental law of creation. This law dictates that to get what you want, you must first give it. Or put another way, what you focus on will expand. There are many ways to employ this law in your life to produce consistent and harmonious results. For instance, if you give with the intention of providing aid or assistance, you will inevitably be provided with more of the same. I'll be talking about this notion more specifically in our discussion of the tools required for working directly with the virtual. For now, simply recognize that all of this is simply another way of looking at the principles discussed earlier concerning attention, intention, desire, and experience.

Through yet another pair of eyes, when you choose the behavior, you choose the consequences. On a practical level, this mechanism can be observed in every human endeavor, from finances to health and gardening to sports. I'm sure you've all been encouraged at one time or another in the sense that, "You can do anything you put your mind to."

■ Identifying Learned Behavior

Usually, though, most of us are simply mimicking learned behavior, at least up until what is popularly called the age of reason. This is meant to infer that at a particular point in your development, you become responsible for your own behavior as the training wheels of the maturing process are removed and you supposedly become capable of making your own decisions and your own choices. Realistically, all you have accomplished by this point is to do what you're told and behave like everyone else in the environment. Freedom of choice is usually limited to continuing to make the choices everyone else has been making for you up until such time.

Nonetheless, this constitutes the environmental aspect of the early maturation process. Subsequently, remnants of these early influences, originating in part from genetics and environment, are woven into the fabric of the real and perceived stresses of becoming responsible for your own outcomes. Once beyond the mandatory supervision of youth, you enter into agreements of choice predicated to a large extent upon the strength of these early influences. Navigating into the deeper waters of adulthood, one can begin to experiment with different choices guided by the results of experiences, cumulative wisdom, and the suggestions that follow.

■ Establishing Priorities

Using the model constructed throughout this book to build the foundation for a new way of being, you'll begin where you are. Understanding that life is tri-dimensional and existence is multidimensional, you recognize that perceptual awareness is communicated through thoughts, feelings, and an overall sense of well-being. In other words, the multidimensional influences that shape experiences are expressed through the tri-dimensional interaction of the physical body, the biochemistry, and the virtual realm.

To effectively change your overall experience in the most productive way, it is necessary that all three of these realms function in sync with each other, rather than working to compensate for imbalances in one or the other realms. It is this out-of-sync compensation that produces chronic low-grade symptoms, which, if left unchecked, eventually degenerate into a diagnosable disease complex. To be more specific, it's time to take a look at some of the practical ways in which you can produce productive changes and restore harmony within and among the realms.

■ Working with the Physical Realm

Although the physical realm is the most readily accessible of the three realms, it often poses the most difficult challenge for people when it comes to altering the way it looks or feels. Fortunately, there are some simple solutions based upon reliable systems that can be easily implemented and maintained with minimal amounts of motivation and consistency. The secondary benefits of addressing concerns in the other realms through the physical realm are equally rewarding. So let's take a look at the three avenues of access for securing physical contentment.

The first is one that everyone does everyday—eat. I'm sure this seems most obvious, and it is. However, it is also one of the most difficult issues for a lot of people. Even if you're entirely motivated to achieve a balanced and optimal alliance with lifestyle changes related to diet, it can be very, very confusing. It seems that everybody has an opinion as to what the optimal diet consists of, how the foods should be selected, prepared and combined, as well as what portions should be eaten and when. To make matters worse, they all seem to contradict each other, while producing variable results at best. But have no fear. You now have the caveats, guidelines, reminders, laws, and suggestions to direct you. Remember, there are no panaceas; everything works; for every action, there is an equal and opposite reaction; and when you hear hoof beats, look for horses.

The first step in the process of determining what's going to work best for you is an assessment of your goals. What do you hope to accomplish with the dietary approach you're considering? Oftentimes, this will simply come down to losing weight. Frequently, feeling good and having more energy are also on the list. Whatever your motivation, remember that the cause of most failure is selecting a system that is flawed. Now this doesn't necessarily mean that the system itself is flawed. It may mean that the system you've selected is inappropriate to your situation or circumstances. Why? Because everything works, but everything works most effectively when it's applied to a given set of circumstances for which it's most indicated.

■ Selecting a System

One of the paradoxes related to this particular issue of diet, is that diets don't work, but you can lose weight on any diet. The question is what type of weight will you lose, how much of it will you lose, how long will it take to lose it, will it last or will you rebound, and is it safe, effective and appropriate for your circumstances?

So the answer to the mystical diet question is simply this: Pick something that fits your lifestyle, because otherwise you will have a difficult time with compliance. Select an approach that contains foods that you like, are easy to find and are simple to prepare; also make sure any approach is flexible enough to accommodate periodic temptations, splurges, and schedule changes. Frankly, you can accomplish any of the common goals of a specific dietary approach with any diet that you are comfortable with and to which you intend to comply.

■ The Rotation Diet

Personally, I'm a big fan of a rotation-type dietary format. I like following different dietary regimens at different points in the year for different periods of time. I do this for a few reasons. It helps prevent boredom and stagnation. It keeps food interesting and helps me to constantly expose myself to different types, kinds, and preparations of the many available food combinations.

Also, it stimulates a natural response in the body called the confusion principle. Simply put, the confusion principle means that when you subject the body to different forms of stimulation, it has to adapt and respond. This usually takes anywhere from three days to two weeks. During this period of time, your metabolism is provoked naturally by the change. Energy levels tend to go up, and your body inevitably sheds some additional pounds because of the alteration in the energy sources being provided to it.

Choosing a Diet

- Find a diet that works for you.
- Adopt a diet that fits your lifestyle.
- Pay attention to cravings and related symptoms.
- Diversify regularly.

So the bottom line is to find a diet that works for you on multiple levels, because you are actually altering relationships within and among the realms at the same time. Also, don't be afraid to diversify. Get creative and try new things.

Now, another important consideration when selecting a dietary approach includes the issue of cravings. These cravings are natural responses by the body and are actually a subtle form of communication. Becoming aware of their significance is an important aspect of choosing what's right for you. These cravings can mean several things, so it's important to pay attention to them and make the necessary adjustments. It's also one of the reasons why it's important to diversify.

■ Understanding Cravings

Cravings can mean that something is lacking in your diet. They can also represent a temporary attempt on the part of your body to adapt to any changes you've introduced. If they last any longer than three weeks, something's wrong. Try including some other varieties of food, or have some nutritional testing performed. Finally, these cravings can be a subtle hint that your eating habits have a heavy emotional overtone, so pay attention.

The reasons you decided to follow a particular dietary approach may indicate that your concerns are rooted in one of the other realms.

■ Five Essential Nutrients

The next essential component of any dietary approach is specific supplementation. Remember earlier that we talked about the five essential nutrients that need to be supplemented everyday? These include a multiple vitamin, a mineral supplement, an antioxidant, digestive enzymes, and probiotics. Beyond these five, if you still have concerns, or are experiencing any diet-related symptoms that last longer than three weeks, it's time to get evaluated with the M.A.P. that I suggested previously.

■ Symptoms and Imbalances

There are a wide variety of possible imbalances that can manifest themselves as symptoms reflecting an even wider variety of possible causes. Properly assessed, these imbalances can be identified, isolated, reversed, eliminated, or managed. If, in fact, the symptoms being experienced are rooted in biochemistry, they can be caused by a simple inequity in supply and demand. But there are a number of other possible, and very common, scenarios that may be represented by the symptoms. For instance, I have personally tested many individuals who for all intents and purposes seem to have constructed an ideal lifestyle while plagued by recurrent symptoms. Oftentimes, these symptoms include everything from joint and muscle pain, to headaches, indigestion, skin rashes, hair loss, constipation, weight gain and insomnia. Frequently, these symptoms merely reflect an imbalance, dysfunction, or deficiency that is simple to remedy once it is identified.

For example, one of the more common scenarios includes a proper diet with supplementation, but there is still an inability to access or adequately digest, transport or assimilate certain specific nutrients. Another example is that of a greater demand for certain nutrients than that being supplied by the diet. This demand may be developed by an excess toxic burden, increased physical activity, or cellular malnutrition provoked by a sedentary lifestyle, insufficient enzyme activity, or inadequate water intake.

■ Integrating Is Essential

Regardless of the symptoms or the cause, developing a comprehensive approach to establishing physical and biochemical well-being must be a primary consideration for directing your efforts, particularly if quality of life is a goal. Considering the fact that close to 80 percent of all degenerative diseases have been linked to diet, the importance of the fuel you select for your physical body cannot be overemphasized. Nutritional testing can be a critical component of refining this approach.

The choices you make regarding the care and feeding of your physical being will directly intersect with your genetic predispositions and learned behaviors. These account for the first two elements of individual susceptibility. However, the third component contributing to what ultimately defines your personal lifestyle is that of stress. As you begin to become proactive in your choices, you begin to see how participation in the process of choosing stresses contributes to creating your overall experience of life.

I saved this next essential element of a comprehensive assessment program for last because it is one of the most difficult for most people to implement and maintain. It ranks second in terms of commitment failures. The final component of a program designed to maintain the integrity of the physical body is that of regular exercise. There, I said it. Now let's talk about it.

■ Exercise Is Critical

Exercise is necessary. Motion is life. The quantity and quality of exercise can be a significant factor in determining the overall effectiveness of any attempt to improve the quality of life. That said, the same rules apply to choosing exercise as apply to selecting a dietary approach. Once you've *given* your attention to the *intention* of exercising, you can use the other tools touched on throughout this book to adopt and refine an approach that will work for you.

The foundation for your program should consist of something that interests you. Choose something that you enjoy, something that you can incorporate and commit to consistently. Once again, anything is better than nothing when it comes to regularly exposing your body to some form of movement, however, there are four characteristics you should look for in any well-rounded approach to exercise.

■ Elements of an Effective Exercise Program

While evaluating potential exercise programs, be sure to look for things that contain elements of strength, flexibility, balance, and endurance. The strength component will ensure a stable ratio of calorie burning lean muscle tissue, while maintaining healthy bone density. Flexibility will help to reduce the accumulation of muscle imbalances, which produce undue structural stresses on the major joints of the body.

Endurance (or cardio) will provide increased oxygen and removal of waste products from all the cells in the body by augmenting circulation. It will also help to accelerate the delivery of vital nutrients, while encouraging the use of stored fat for energy. Most importantly, it will increase your resistance to heart attacks and strokes by strengthening your cardiovascular system. Additional benefits include a reduction in food cravings, improvement in hormonal balance, increased energy, and a well-toned, aesthetically pleasing, lean physique.

Balance will help to provide stimulation to the fine stabilizing muscle groups that tend to be ignored during daily activities and routine exercise programs. Stimulating these muscle groups will contribute to equilibrium and coordination. Functional muscle strength will improve such that your activities of daily living can be performed with ease.

All of these goals can be achieved with some combination of interval training and strength training. As always, changing your routine periodically will discourage boredom while encouraging gains in vitality, energy, mood enhancement, and sleep. The laws governing exercise physiology

Remember . . .

- Motion is life.
- Exercise is essential.
- Choose something you like and can commit to.
- Cross-train regularly.
- Look for exercise that combines flexibility, strength, balance, and endurance.
- Take time to relax and recover.

are universal and can be applied to anyone's situation, regardless of age or current physical condition. They just need to be adapted to your *specific set of circumstances.*

■ The Benefits of Walking

Perhaps one of the simplest and most beneficial of all possible exercise choices is that of walking. Remember, one of the goals in developing a comprehensive program for longevity is the greatest return for the least investment. If a little voice says, "Go for a walk," it might be your brain telling you what it needs.

Two studies reveal how the simple act of taking a walk each day may offer significant protection from a major health problem. Cognitive decline is a symptom that signals the possible onset of Alzheimer's disease (the leading cause of dementia among aging adults). *The Journal of the American Medical Association* published two studies that address the effects of light exercise on cognitive decline in older women and dementia in elderly men.

Harvard researchers conducted the first study. Questionnaires were used to assess physical activity levels and exercise patterns for more than 18,700 women, aged seventy to eighty-one years. Questionnaires covered a minimum of nine years, and were followed up with two telephone interviews with each subject to assess cognitive health measures, such as memory and attention span.

Researchers noted much better cognitive function and less cognitive decline were both strongly associated with "long-term regular physical activity, including walking." They found that women who walked two to three hours at an easy pace each week "performed significantly better on these tests of cognition than women who walked less than one hour per week." Even less cognitive decline was noted in women who walked six or more hours each week. These results parallel another benefit of regular walking among women.

A previous six-year breast cancer study that included data on more than 74,000 women over the age of fifty, found that women who exercise regularly have lower breast cancer rates. Only a couple of hours of brisk walking each week may provide enough exercise to reduce breast cancer risk. The second study looked at the association between walking exercise and the risk of dementia in men aged seventy-one to ninety-three. They collected three years of exercise data on more than 2,200 men. At the outset of the study, none of the men had been diagnosed with dementia or conditions that would prevent them from walking (like stroke or Parkinson's disease). Over several years, two follow-up exams were conducted to assess neurological health. Almost 160 of the men developed dementia during the study period. Results show that men who walked between a quarter mile and one mile per day had a lower risk of dementia than those who walked less than a quarter mile each day. In this study, more was clearly better because men who walked less than a quarter mile per day had nearly *twice* the risk of dementia, compared to those who walked more than two miles each day.

■ Why Does This Work?

What is it about taking a daily walk that might prevent cognitive decline and dementia? It could have something to do with cholesterol's association to Alzheimer's disease. Previous research has suggested that high cholesterol levels may increase the level of a certain protein that is abnormally processed by people with Alzheimer's disease. This abnormal processing sets off a chain reaction that causes a peptide to accumulate and form tangles that can kill brain cells.

A Georgetown University Medical Center study showed how high cholesterol levels significantly increase the rate at which these tangles are formed. In addition, the researchers concluded that high cholesterol also increases the production of a different protein that transports cholesterol out of the cell. And while that's a normal function, in this situation, it results in an unfortunate increase of free cholesterol, which has a toxic effect on nerve cells.

Of course, daily exercise is one of the best and safest ways to control cholesterol levels. None of the researchers speculated on why regular exercise through walking might have helped prevent cognitive decline and dementia, but it seems likely that reducing cholesterol levels may have come into play. Remember, the functional integrity of the nervous system is dictated by use, not age. Furthermore, the simple process of nutrients in and waste products out maintains the viability of these and every cell in every system of the body.

Now, if it seems I'm being a bit vague at this point, I am. I've done this intentionally because the specific application of the principles governing each realm will differ from person to person and situation to situation. Remember, everything works, and there are no panaceas. However, there are some universal guidelines that apply to everyone and every realm. I have consolidated these into a cheat sheet summary in the appendix at the end of this book. For the moment, let's proceed through a similarly broad overview of the other two realms, beginning with the transitional world of biochemistry.

■ Working with the Biochemical Realm

Because the biochemical realm is bi-directional, it provides for and responds to stimulation from the other two realms. The biochemical realm influences and is influenced more obviously than the other two realms, simply because it is more accessible and easier to monitor objectively. It is rare to find a primary imbalance rooted in the biochemical realm unless it is related to a genetic malfunction. It is possible, however, to create an imbalance in this realm, which occurs primarily due to repetitive or cumulative assaults on the other two realms.

More commonly, you see symptoms arising in the biochemical realm that are subtle, chronic, and undetectable with conventional assessments. This system is the most responsive to intervention in a Vicious Cycle Disorder. It usually begins to express itself in the form of symptoms as a result of functional imbalances or supply-demand problems. Once detected, manipulating dietary protocols and supplying specific supplementation usually easily resolve these discrepancies.

Compliance with a system that works is critical when attempting to resolve issues involving human biochemistry. This is one of the reasons for vagueness when it comes to specific dietary approaches and the nature of specific supplementation. In addition to the supplemental foundational nutrients discussed in the overview of diet, there are a myriad of possible needs that arise in every system of the body, which are unique from person to person, and scenario to scenario. These are called therapeutic enhancements, and can only be identified through assessment of one's individual biochemical environment.

■ Begin with Biochemistry

Because of the tremendous overlap with the other two realms, and the unique accessibility of the biochemistry for evaluation, it is frequently a good starting point for assessing an approach to realm integration. This territory can be easily monitored and is highly suggestive in terms of establishing contributory relationships between causes and symptoms.

The biochemical realm can also easily serve as a springboard for identifying the cause of symptoms originating in the other two realms. If a symptom is rooted in the biochemical realm, the biochemistry, and the associated symptoms, will typically improve when treated through the biochemistry. Similarly treated, if the symptoms are primarily rooted in one of the other realms, the biochemistry will usually improve, but the symptoms will not. Again, there are exceptions to every rule, but generally these broad guidelines will apply. Regardless, an assessment of the biochemical environment is a cornerstone for objectively identifying causal factors, particularly if a dysfunction is suspected in any tissue, organ, gland, or system.

■ Significance of the G.I. Tract

With the gastrointestinal tract being the hub of activity for imbalances originating in the biochemical realm, evaluation of suspicious symptoms can usually be quickly associated with a cause. However, all too often, this is where the journey begins and ends. Very little consideration is given to the possibility that the presenting symptoms are being caused by problems in one of the other realms. More often, if the symptoms are expressed through a particular system, the search for a cause is limited to that system. If a cause is not obvious, the symptoms are treated and realm compensation begins to occur. If what the body is attempting to communicate is not heard, it will endeavor to correspond in some other manner. So the hoof beats are heard, but since the horses aren't found, attempts to drown out the sound of the hoof beats are initiated.

Granted, the gastrointestinal tract is a very important conduit to all of the realms. From a functional perspective, it is responsible for harnessing energy that enables growth, repair, reproduction, and the proliferation of life. The everyday jobs in this system include digesting foods, absorbing and assimilating nutrients, and eliminating waste products from the body. Obviously, these primary functions are essential elements to the quality of life for any living organism. And it is exactly for this reason that a fundamental awareness of the care and nurturing of this critical system must be integrated into any self-directed wellness initiative.

Fostering a productive biochemical environment can be especially challenging, given the dual nature of its functional relationship with the other realms, and the daily assaults on its integrity. Conversely, similar to the physical realm, there are some variables that can be manipulated to minimize the cumulative effects of micro-trauma produced by exposure to the technological trauma of modern day society. Innocent enough in small doses, repeated contact with environmental pollutants, food additives, solar radiation, and other sources of toxic stress can cause the biochemistry to shift into a compensatory defense mode that produces vague wide-spread symptoms indistinguishable from primary disease entities.

■ The Usual Suspects

In addition to the freedom to choose what you eat and drink, you can also scrutinize your interactions with other known adversaries. Some of these are obvious, some less so. In the obvious category, you can monitor your fluid intake, your dietary choices, the types of medications you take, the amount of exercise you engage in, and your exposure to environmental toxins.

In the not-so-obvious category, you can become aware of some of the pitfalls associated with the obvious items. You can also explore some of the hidden potential hazards associated with things you have assumed are relatively safe. You are, no doubt, at risk with every aspect of decision-making that involves what you eat, drink, inhale, see, touch, feel, and think.

The "trade-offs" for the convenience of modern day living are well touted. In fact, they are so well publicized that you might tend to take them for granted to the extent that you have become desensitized to their deadly promise. The toxic by-products of contemporary convenience are generally classified as xenobiotics, which are defined as completely synthetic compounds that do not naturally occur on the earth. The only common thread among xenobiotics is that they are foreign to the human body. This includes an array of chemicals including pharmaceutical residues, endocrine-disrupting chemicals, personal care products, food additives, preservatives, and pesticides. The significance of these compounds is their potential for adverse health effects, interaction with other compounds, and results of low-level chronic exposure. With the advent of the information highway, it is becoming easier to become educated about these potential consequences. Conversely, because of the fast food consciousness that permeates our collective environment, it is also easier to reflexively subscribe to a relationship with these "healthy imposters" than with the multidimensional influences of mindful choice. Nonetheless, just because you are surrounded by a myriad of choices doesn't mean that you can't make informed decisions. The journey toward change is initiated through an awareness of the new questions that lead toward new actions or behaviors.

■ Pick a Path

For instance, I am often asked for guidance in dealing with a particular issue, such as excess weight, chronic pain, acid reflux, headaches, or menopause. Obviously, a choice has been made at some point to seek counsel beyond the advice offered in the onslaught of remedies proposed in media advertisements. Part of the initial exploration employed in a search for the cause of these symptoms is often a list of partial strategies. This list is designed to engage the participant in further investigation beyond the office visit. Frequently, this list is simply a group of words that represent universal influences to which everyone is subjected to in the physical realm. It is intended to provoke a general awareness of common influences in an individual's routine environment.

These influences are generally arranged into two categories. These categories include things in the daily environment that may be contributing to individual concerns, and things that may be readily available in that same environment to assist in resolving those concerns. The first list usually contains generic items that are known to be widespread and harmful. These are things like sugar, caffeine, alcohol, fried foods, etc. Of course, there are also some more specific things on the list that require a little more investigation on the part of the participant, but that's really the point of this approach.

The other list contains equally simple tools for exploration with a different focus. It contains things that are equally widespread and available, and that are known to be productive substitutes for the items in the other list. They may simply be alternatives to the choices that contributed to the problem that brought the person to my office. These include things that they may be unaware of that they could easily alter their exposure to without tremendous difficulty. In other words, these are alternative choices that they can make that will contribute to resolving the problem instead of perpetuating it, such as dietary alternatives that might improve digestion and reduce the need for expensive medications, increased intake of water, reducing consumption of candy, ice cream, white bread, highly processed snack foods with chemical additives, and soda pop. Simple substitutes might be to increase the fruits, vegetables, and whole grain foods that provide the nutrients they need.

By executing this type of inventory, a number of potentially productive processes are initiated. For one, the patient has been offered another way to look at things. This individual is also supplied with a streamlined (although partial and generic) list of suggestions for altering their own experience. The immediate goal here is to create awareness and to substitute behaviors.

Persons who choose to act upon this information often return with additional questions based upon their experimentation. They frequently experience dramatic progress in their condition by virtue of the changes they have implemented. So with the simple cataloging of some commonly used words, a life is changed simply by participation. That individual has become proactive by virtue of the choices they have selected to implement and begun to accept responsibility for their situation in life.

■ Something to Chew On

Our technologically advanced society sometimes seems engorged with choices to help simplify our lives. Or is it? Take, for example, the choice to use a microwave oven for preparing meals. It's quick, simple, easy ... and dangerous to your health. Dangerous because the trade-off for quick, simple and easy is a heating process that increases cholesterol, increases white blood cell numbers, decreases red blood cell numbers, and causes a depletion and mutation of the nutrients in a given food. This, in turn, produces compounds that are unknown in nature called radiolytic compounds.

When evaluating current lifestyle choices, other examples of "food for thought items" on the list of things to consider might range from the obvious to the seemingly obscure. This may include things such as: How much sleep do you get? Do you exercise regularly? What type of exercise do you perform? How long do you exercise? How much sugar do you consume daily? Do you drink caffeinated beverages? Do you drink carbonated beverages? How much and how many of each do you consume daily? Do you take regular vacations? How often do you take them and how long do you stay? Do you have a particular spiritual belief? Do you experience any of the following symptoms regularly, i.e. depression, indigestion, headaches, nightmares, insomnia, constipation, joint pain, etc.? Do you hold a particular belief regarding any of the following, i.e., cholesterol causes heart disease, an aspirin a day can reduce your risk of heart attack, additional calcium can stop bone loss, etc.?

The point of such a survey is to establish a basis for understanding where the resistance, obstacles, or contributing factors to symptom complexes in an individual lifestyle might reside. As a result, the initial set of recommendations for any given individual can be constructed in such a fashion as to work more closely with established behaviors and beliefs, while encouraging gentle shifts in perception and patterns of activities. Typically, this makes the recommendations more specific and more palatable, while increasing the likelihood of compliance and follow-through.

Often, simple modifications in established patterns of behavior can result in dramatic and productive changes in moods, attitudes, and an overall feeling of well-being. Suggestions, such as take time to eat, chew your food thoroughly, increase your water intake, increase your intake of vegetables, increase your intake of grains, eat ripe fruit in season, decrease your intake of animal products, or drink minimal fluids with your meals, can go a long way toward improving low-grade feelings of fatigue or indigestion.

■ Facing Facts

Finally, creating awareness through some non-challenging and non-confrontational facts can serve to increase awareness and change counterproductive behaviors without threatening, judging, or embarrassing a motivated individual. These facts might include some simple declarations in the form of educational instructions. These instructions can incorporate concepts, such as the dangers of processed foods, depleted food sources resulting from depleted soils, overcooking foods with heat above 118 degrees, which destroys active enzymes and denatures proteins, etc. This might even be expanded to offer simple, but encouraging, advice for seeking alternatives, such as most of the foods that you eat should not need a label (If man made it, don't eat it), or avoid any food with ingredients listed on the label that you can't pronounce.

In this way, it is possible to offer an individual another way of looking at things, which has traditionally been offered as advice in other forms, such as avoid processed, pasteurized, pre-packaged, and flash-frozen foods; or avoid foods with additives, chemical preservatives, or artificial colors. Regardless of how the information is communicated or received, the net impact will always be a change in awareness. From that standpoint, it will make more sense and offer more encouragement in recognizing that there are viable alternatives that don't require a cloistered lifestyle.

At times, sharing some simple facts concerning the reality of an established behavior pattern will suffice to energize a new dynamic in an individual's life. For instance, at times I've found it appropriate to simply state the fact that the food industry lobby has established legislation that allows commercial food manufacturers to *not* list approximately 15,000 additives on the labels of grocery store foods.

To emphasize the importance of this established practice in a high-risk individual, I might add that the inclusion of these substances has been demonstrated to produce predictable consequences in anyone who routinely consumes these chemical-laden food substances. Those consequences include cravings for that particular food, potential addiction to that food, making you fat, making you hungry, and contributing to heart disease and cancer by virtue of the concentration of trans fatty acids. The nature of the initial advice and recommendations depends to a large degree upon where an individual is starting. If the afflicted individual is desperate, they will do anything. If their symptoms are chronic and low-grade, but tolerable, where they are being asked to go may be too far to travel from where they presently dwell.

■ Start with a Checklist

Initially, a simple checklist of things to monitor may suffice and may be all that they can handle at that point in time. If so, a simple page of recommended do's and don'ts is all that is needed. This might include a minimal, but specific, list of things to begin including and things to begin avoiding. For the purpose of supporting health and longevity, the best advice for any initial lifestyle change involving diet is to eat fresh, whole, high quality, unprocessed foods. This includes recommendations for minimizing or eliminating artificial sweeteners, artificial flavors, artificial preservatives, artificial colors, or hydrogenated oils. In general, one of the easiest ways to begin the transition to a healthy lifestyle is to avoid products with added sugars, including desserts, soft drinks, and snacks. Although fresh fruit juice is a wholesome beverage, it is best consumed in small quantities or diluted to minimize its concentrated sweetness.

If this sounds like a lot of work, it can be. It depends upon where you are when you start, and what kind of resources you bring to the table in the form of experience, exposure, awareness, and receptivity. Nonetheless, this is the challenge at hand. While I am not suggesting that you substitute my opinion for your own, I am suggesting that if you are experiencing recurrent concerns, you consider another way of looking at the advice that you have chosen to follow. In the final analysis, the instructions you choose to follow will determine the future you will create.

■ Recognize Partial Truths

Now, this is not to say that I have all the answers or even any answers. The point is more suggestive of the fact that everyone has something to offer because everything works. Everyone is in possession of the truth, or more correctly, a truth or an aspect of the truth. These partial truths are part of the influences from which you have to choose in constructing your own path through life.

One of the dangers at this point is to assume that someone else can solve your problem. This is dangerous because the individual seen as the problem-solver begins to believe that they have some special gift. It is also risky because the individual seeking advice may begin to substitute the opinion of the problem-solver for his or her own opinion. This is not the point of this interaction. The point is simply to provide a catalyst for change based upon the suggestion of someone who is more experienced with a particular process. It is primarily instructive and designed for redirecting the footsteps of the person who is looking for another way to get where they want to go.

■ Two Sources of Influence

The influences affecting the condition of an afflicted individual generally emerge from two sources. One is contrived and constructed. These primarily impact one's day-to-day experience. Therefore, they comprise one aspect of our tri-dimensional nature to the extent that you choose to interact with them and subscribe to their influence. They include all of the things that you choose to become involved with in the form of activities and routine behaviors.

The other set of influences contribute to the multidimensional nature of existence. Unless you are sensory-impaired, you are routinely and unavoidably subjected to these persuasive temptations. They are designed to motivate us to act, encourage us to repeat behavior, and seduce us into submitting to a relationship that temporarily, but repeatedly, gratifies a need or produces a satisfying stimulation of our senses. These influences are the result of random exposure to the people, places, and things in our surroundings that are generated and perpetuated beyond our conscious control.

In addition to temperature effects, subtle influences may be significantly generated by changes in relative humidity or even ambient light, causing you to feel differently for no apparent reason. A common source of externally induced influence is produced by magnetic fields that can also affect the way that you feel. Acoustical noise can be quite difficult to characterize and test but the influences on the mind can be both heard and seen. An example of this is when someone is talking to you. You consciously perceive or understand what that person is saying to you. Another example is when you look at a movie. You see the characters portrayed, the action and anything else the eye and ear can see and hear. This type of influence on our minds is called conscious perception.

There is another type of perception known as subliminal or subconscious perception. This type of perception deals with the ability of the brain to process a message without the person being aware of what is being processed. Can we sense stimuli that are below our absolute thresholds and consciously perceiving something? The answer is clearly yes. Can we be affected by stimuli too weak for us ever to notice? Recent experiments hint that, under certain conditions, the answer may again be yes. It is a subliminal message because you are not consciously aware of it, for instance, when a song is played. The music, the words, even the combination of instruments, can be used to provoke certain, feelings, emotions, memories, and visual images. None of this occurs consciously, but your brain still processes it!

So, we can process information without being aware of it. A weak stimulus triggers a weak response within us—a response that may reach our brain where it evokes a feeling, even though we may not be consciously aware of the stimulus. What the conscious mind can't recognize, the heart may know.

A subliminal message is delivered to the brain without the person being aware of its existence or that it was sent. A subliminal message bypasses the "mental defenses" (the RAS system) of the conscious mind of your awareness and is delivered to the brain as it is. Therefore, our minds *can* sense subliminal messages even though we are not aware of their presence.

One aspect of these subtle multidimensional influences is to a certain extent contrived in that you choose where to go, how to get there, who to see, and what to do. But what happens once you are in a certain environment is really a function of the influences contributing to that environment. All of the sights, sounds, smells, attitudes, personalities, and activities present in any given environment will generate influences to which you are exposed by virtue of your choice to attend and participate.

The overriding feature that distinguishes them from the more natural tri-dimensional influences is the element of a conscious choice. A three-dimensional experience is provoked by the choice to indulge or engage in it. For the most part you know what you will be exposed to when you decide to go to a party, a theme park, the beach, a museum, or an opera. The multidimensional aspect of this experience is produced by all the other people and things that comprise the environment. These are the things you experience beyond your physical presence in the environment in which these other forms of stimuli exist. This means that you may not even be aware of the fact that you are choosing to be exposed to some of them. Examples would be the effects of exposure to toxins in the environment, such as the air you breathe, the water you drink, and different types of invisible waves in the sound and light spectrums. Even the dominant belief systems, social mores, or prevalent socialized behavior of a particular society, although partially contrived, produce an unspoken and unseen sphere of influence that is felt and responded to on some level.

Despite the fact that you may have chosen a lifestyle with which you are comfortable, you surely become aware of a related unspoken disapproval when you enter an environment in which the way that you look, think, act, dress, or behave produces a "tension so thick you could cut it with a knife." This is the nature of the subtle influences that comprise the multidimensional experiences of existence.

■ Contrived Influences

The contrived set of influences consists of things that you come into contact with everyday and that represent life's smorgasbord menu. It includes things like which TV channels and shows you submit your senses to on a regular basis. It also includes the foods you select to eat, how you choose to prepare them, what medications you take on a regular basis, what type of exercise you choose to engage in, the type of work you perform, where you choose to spend your money, the types of supplements you take, the newspapers and magazines you read, how you spend your free time, and the type of recreation in which you engage. In other words, it is comprised of all of the influences you select to submit yourself to that you have direct and immediate access to and control of in terms of the choices you make.

> **A Three-Legged Stool**
>
> ■ Life is tri-dimensional.
> ■ Existence is multidimensional.
> ■ An imbalance in one realm creates imbalance in the others.
> ■ Diseases are symptoms of an undiagnosed imbalance.

The patterns of behavior that emerge as a result of exposure to these influences play a large role in determining the types of tri-dimensional life experiences you will have. Most of these interactions can be changed, modified, or in some other way altered to impact the quality of life you experience. They are also at the root of most of the problems and concerns that accumulate to express themselves as imbalances in any of the three realms.

More often, the choices you make from this menu are directly linked to the more subtle influences of genetics, environment, and stress. Nonetheless, if engaged in routinely (or unconsciously), they form into patterns of habits that dictate your physical experience by contributing to pressure thresholds in one of the realms. This culmination of events is typically the cause of the chronic low-grade discomfort you experience that ultimately leads you to seek help from a professional caregiver.

Unfortunately, unless a whole person perspective is employed as part of evaluating the concerns these thresholds represent, all too often, this is just the beginning of an endless stream of frustrating attempts to associate the experience of symptoms with an active disease process. The result is usually a prescription for the symptoms, since the test results return as normal, but the discomfort persists.

■ Self-Induced Stress

The reality is that discomfort originates as a result of the cumulative effects produced by your choices. Initially, these effects merely produce a constant sense of awareness that something is not right. This awareness is necessarily indistinct at this stage, since it only represents an attempt by your body to communicate a concern. It also suggests that its innate capacity to respond to some excessive demand is being challenged, and its ability to compensate is being taxed. This represents the true nature of a Vicious Cycle Disorder.

Interacting with someone experiencing symptoms at this stage is most demanding, most rewarding, most difficult, and most productive. Since everything is what it isn't, and the solution is always in the problem, adopting a different way of looking at things will usually provide a change in what is seen. Subsequent changes also occur in how one responds, what is recommended, and what is produced.

It is at this point that a lifestyle assessment is most essential and productive. It is also the point at which the "everything works" caveat is most compelling. In fact, conventional testing to rule out diagnosable disease actually provides the benefit of pointing out the direction of the most probable cause of concerns by ruling out what it is not. The challenge at this juncture is to move beyond the negative test results into another way of looking at things, rather than waiting to see something familiar in the way things are routinely observed.

■ No News Is Good News

For example, an individual may present him or herself with any of an infinite number of usual symptomatic concerns involving an expression of discomfort in the physical body. This person may be visibly disturbed and frustrated with the absence of positive findings to explain his or her distress. Having ruled out an obvious disease process as the cause of the concerns doesn't necessarily rule out a process as the cause of their symptoms. Using the "hoof beats and horses" caveat, one can quickly move on to a broader assessment of behavior patterns and lifestyle choices to identify the underlying imbalances that are contributing to the undiagnosed symptoms.

In fact, more benefit is to be had in a productive assessment at this level than in attempting to treat a process that has already progressed to the status of a diagnosable disease. Since anything can cause anything, and there are no panaceas, the likelihood of actually "curing" a disease is highly improbable. However, the possibility of altering patterns of behavior to effect a change in the experience of undiagnosable symptoms is far more likely.

The fact is that conventional medicine does not presently incorporate, nor give much credence to, whole person or lifestyle assessment. This undoubtedly will change as the flawed system currently in place fails to respond to the demands of an ailing population, and greater numbers of unresolved symptom complexes begin to plague the masses. In the meantime, you must each continue to work on yourselves as a contribution to the subtle sphere of multidimensional influences populating the experience of existence. Remember, one of the fundamental laws governing conscious creation is that you get what you give. Ultimately, there is justice and, therefore, promise and hope. Our faith, then, is truly the substance of things hoped for and the evidence of things not yet seen.

■ Reconciling the Unseen Realm

As you continue to construct a practical working model to accompany you through your life experiences, a return to the unseen realm is imminent. Having peered through different eyes at the physical and biochemical realms, perhaps a different pair of glasses will assist in seeing the unseen as a viable tool for consciously manifesting the life of your dreams.

The core operating system of this realm is fueled by information and energy. These paired resources are accessed in large part by your expectations. In fact, 90 percent of manifestation is expectation. So, what keeps you from consciously manifesting what you truly desire? Well, given the nature of this realm, the answer is simpler than you might think. The other 10 percent of manifestation is evoked by the words you speak. One of the key techniques for accelerating conscious manifestation is to observe the words that you speak. In so doing, you will be able to identify the potential source of repeated experiences and how to use words as an access to the virtual.

The virtual realm also presents itself as a unique paradox in that it is unseen. It is also the least explored or considered when evaluating the status of a physical condition. Yet, in reality, it is the most straightforward and easiest to understand and operate. But it is also the source of most, if not all, of the problems, concerns, and self-imposed obstacles preventing you from experiencing the desires of your heart. To truly understand and appreciate the impact and relationship of this realm to the other two, a brief digression to the bi-directional function of the biochemical realm is indicated.

■ Bi-Directional Benefits

As you remember, the biochemical realm is bi-directional in that it communicates both to and from the unseen realm. It also directly interacts with the physical in the same capacity. It carries vital nutrients, information, and waste products to and from every system in the body. But, it is because of its direct communication with the virtual that it becomes such a valuable tool for assessing causal relationships with symptoms.

In the discussion of the biochemical realm, a theoretical model was constructed involving communication pathways existing between the virtual and the physical. Recall that the anatomical pathways of biochemistry demonstrate the mechanisms by which events occur, but do not suggest the manner by which they originate.

■ Past, Future, Now

As attention is directed toward one of the two groups in which the character of thought resides, a reaction occurs. Bear in mind these two groups of thoughts are represented by past guilt and future anxiety. However, you experience each in the present moment of awareness. This experience is brought forth from the virtual through the biochemical into the physical by small particles of matter. These particles characterize the underlying feeling or emotion associated with the experience. The experience originates in the nature of the thoughts routinely entertained. The subsequent behavior is the reaction to the thoughts manifested as a physical expression.

■ Focus Causes Expansion

Applying the model for manifestation to this scenario, you can see how it works. Understand that 90 percent of manifestation is expectation, and that you dwell in one of the two groups above (past guilt or future anxiety) comprising the pool of approximately 60,000 daily thoughts. Since what is focused on expands, the mere act of repeatedly directing attention toward one of the two groups of thoughts produces the intention of experiencing what attention is directed toward.

Expecting to experience a particular event in a particular way is the driving force behind the resulting mechanism of manifestation from the virtual to the physical. The expectation focuses attention toward an intention. The intention cascades from the unseen through the biochemical conduit of molecules, which, in turn, stimulate the creative machinery built into the DNA to materialize the desired result.

■ The Cause of All Causes

Looking at Vicious Cycle Disorders from this perspective unveils a most devious variation of the theme—that of Repetitive Thought Disorders. This may, in fact, be the cause of all causes. Nonetheless, it is of little value if you are unable to access the core mechanism and alter it in some productive way. Thus, the goal becomes thinking new thoughts. To accomplish this effectively and efficiently, a practice must be adopted by which the various attributes of this dynamic are engaged. But first, these attributes must be identified.

Appraising the principal inventory of this virtual manifestation machine, information, energy, attention, intention, thoughts, words, and experiences are found. Delving a bit further, memories, choices, senses, emotions, feelings, imaginings and actions are discovered. As I stated early on, memories of the past fuel the desire for future experiences. The actions you choose produce these subsequent experiences. These experiences create desires to either repeat or avoid the results of a choice, and to perform in a particular manner.

■ Everyone Manifests

Before proceeding, it is important to recognize that everyone manifests, or turns thoughts into things. Therefore, thoughts are things. The word manifest comes from the Middle English word "manifestus," which means visible. It is also derived from the Latin word "manus," which means hand. So one could conclude that in manifesting, you metaphorically reach into the realm of your thoughts with the hand of your words to bring them into existence, making them part of your experience. Another way of looking at this might be that experience is the fruit of seeds planted as thoughts, which are nourished with words.

In sorting out the entire inventory of unique characteristics associated with this primary realm of creative influences, the goal is straightforward. You want to organize these items in a way that directly contributes to your conscious ability to employ them consistently and effectively in creating a reality that productively satisfies and fulfills. To do so, further assigning them to categories of cause and effect is helpful. It quickly becomes apparent that memories, senses, emotions, feelings, intentions, imaginings, desires, expectations, and experiences are a direct result of choices, actions, words, and thoughts.

■ Manifesting from Source

Therefore, you can construct your approach to conscious manifestation on the framework of these four primary operating systems. Your thoughts lead to choices that result in words and actions, which create expectation, attention, intention, and manifestation. Upon additional inspection of the four factors directly contributing to the manifestation of experience, you will find a functional relationship that further assists in defining a core operating system. It seems that choices and actions share the dual influences of cause and effect. Part of the reason you continue to engage them is based upon prior experience. Therefore, you come back to thoughts and words as the source of grist for the mill of conscious manifestation.

Unlike the more loosely structured programs available for altering our physical and biochemical experiences, the applications selected for actively working in the virtual realm will have a more profound and immediate impact upon your day-to-day experiences. This is true simply because there are far fewer choices in terms of things to manipulate to modify your creation. Despite the fact that the virtual is comprised of energy and information, thoughts and words will dictate how they are constructed and what they will symbolize in terms of tangible life experiences.

■ Conscious Creation

Of course, you may choose to allow this mechanism to operate in random response to the fundamental influences of genetics, environment, and stresses. Or you may simply be content to allow yourself to repeatedly be victimized by past choices and future anxieties. However, one of the goals of this book is to erect a working model that provides a productive, predictable, and consistent method for consciously creating the life of your dreams. In fact, by simply adopting some of the suggestions associated with modifying your behavior in the physical and biochemical realms, you are already employing some of these concepts. In pursuing a relationship with the virtual, you are seeking access to the fundamental operating system of creation.

And so, in deconstructing the key elements of the unseen, you are confronted with your thoughts and words. Since your words fertilize the seeds of your thoughts, let's begin with

Thinking about Thoughts

- You have 60,000 thoughts per day.
- The majority of thoughts are the same day after day.
- All thoughts arise in the present moment.
- Many thoughts are about past guilt and future anxiety.
- The space between thoughts is the soil for new thoughts.
- The nature of our thoughts will determine our life experience.
- Repetitive Thought Disorders produce VCD.
- VCD are repeated patterns of behavior.

the seeds you plant and see if there is a way to enrich the soil of your life experience. The raw materials, or core elements, of the soil exist as pure consciousness. However, they must be nourished and nurtured to express their best qualities. Since this soil is essentially composed of information and energy, you will first need to cultivate this soil to prepare it for the seeds.

The tools for accomplishing this consist of attention and intention. Attention activates the vital apparatus of the energy component of the soil, and intention energizes the information component. Both are essential for transformation of the soil of the unseen into a highly receptive medium for the manifestation of your desires. In no realm is it truer that you reap what you sow than in the realm of the virtual.

Superficial applications of this principle appear repeatedly in everyday experiences. But you have developed selective receptivity to outside stimuli as a means of compensating for the sheer volume of influences vying for your attention. And why do they vie? Remember, we're not the only ones who have figured out that attention creates the intention to experience. When's the last time you bought a lime green car only to see hundreds of them on the road after your purchase? There's a reason they call us consumers. What have you consumed today? Now, on to the seeds you sow.

■ Virtual Anatomy

Before examining the ways available for consciously interacting with the operating system of the virtual, you must appraise exactly what you are attempting to interact with. So, let's start with the gross anatomy before considering the physiology of this realm. Well known at this point are the best guess estimates of the 60,000 thoughts entertained each day. It has also been proposed that part of the problem in manipulating the hardwired mechanisms of this system is that the same 60,000 thoughts are entertained everyday. Assuming both of these to be true, a quick look at the possibilities and goals is fitting. After all, what have you got to lose? If your best thinking got you where you are, then if you don't like what comes as a result of changing your approach, you can always go back to your previous behavior.

If thoughts are the seeds of experiences, and the bulk of daily thinking is consumed by thoughts of past experiences and future worries, is it any wonder that your present moments are riddled with turmoil and anxiety? Herein, lie the problem and the solution. Before you can implement change, you must first recognize that change is necessary. You must also determine where and how to apply it.

Obviously, the goal at this stage would be to recognize the types of thoughts that regularly compete for your attention and attempt to change them, eliminate them, substitute them, or at least have fewer of them. The ultimate goal here is to access the core operating system of conscious man-ifestation and employ it to create exactly what you really want. Remember, the first step is to know where you are. Knowing where you want to go is the next step, and knowing how to get there is the final step. So one of the more obvious objectives at this stage might be to identify what it is that you want. The simple act of identifying what you want is the first step in the process of getting it.

■ Tending Your Garden

The long and short of this process is that, if you can consider your thoughts to be the garden from which the nature and quality of your existence will ultimately be determined, then acquiring the tools to effectively tend to that garden will become a priority in your life. Once you begin to devote your attention to where you are, you will begin to form intentions as to how you want to nurture your future development.

All of the rest of the tools and techniques for accomplishing this uncomplicated matter are based upon this one simple realization. Every-thing else is simply a refinement of the various traits, characteristics and attributes associated with the quality and quantity of your experience. But without this first step, random access is all that you will ever be entitled to experience, because everything is based upon this cause set in motion. As Einstein said, "Nothing happens until something moves." As with the approaches to the other realms, once awareness is piqued, the rest is simply a matter of choosing, experimenting, and remaining flexible, creative, receptive, and committed. That's right, pick something that you're comfort-able with, that you enjoy, that produces tangible results, and with which you can remain consistent. There is no reason that working with the virtual and creating from nothing can't be fun. Actually, in my experience, it's far more fun than working with the other two realms.

■ Virtual Access

There are two major pathways for approaching the dynamic of conscious interaction with the virtual. One is simply recognizing that because you are born of the same essence that creates and sustains all of reality, you are, in fact, that essence. Therefore, there really is nothing to do but relax, observe, and enjoy. This is based in large part upon the earlier discussion of spirit. If spirit is universal consciousness, and there is no where that spirit is ever not, then this present moment is a perfect opportunity to observe that which is being experienced by the spirit that exists in you.

> **More Words of Wisdom**
>
> ■ The main thing that's wrong is that you think something's wrong.
> ■ Nothing happens until something moves.
> ■ Successful results depend on desire, commitment, and a system that works.
> ■ You are ultimately responsible for everything you experience.

Because everything is what it isn't, this is both the simplest and most difficult path to travel, since it involves a journey from where most people currently experience life to the present moment in which life is being experienced. Obviously, neither the past nor the future is now. However, your thoughts about both occur in the present moment. Therefore, you are in effect experiencing the life you expect based upon the focused intention of the thoughts you choose right now, creating the future events that will comprise your life in the next moments of your existence.

The other major pathway of access to a present-moment consciousness is that of adopting specific and consistent practices designed to lead you into a place where you can recognize that the thoughts you entertain concerning the past and future exist here and now. This path paradoxically is the easiest to initiate, yet more difficult to sustain, because of the constant interaction with distraction. Nonetheless, there are some practical ways in which this approach might be used to assist in creating a conscious experience of life.

■ Reconstructing Your Thought Database

The most accessible starting point is the 60,000 daily thought database and the allocation of those thoughts into past and future. The immediate goal is to employ a technique that allows for a reconstruction of the database from which your worldly experiences originate. There are two major pathways of access for accomplishing this goal.

The first is by observing the mechanism by which you bring forth those thoughts into your conscious experience—that of your words. This technique is simple and readily available because you use words repeatedly to express your wants, desires, expectations, fears, doubts, and imaginings. The character and content of the words you speak strongly suggest the nature of the thoughts associated with them. So, if you're interested in assessing the status of your thought pool, start with examining the words you most frequently speak.

If your conversation is wrought with words that convey lack, insecurity, anger, discontent, or any of a host of other counterproductive concepts, you have just identified a significant potential cause for your routine experiences. You have also recognized an equally valuable solution. That which you focus on expands, so change your focus and change your experience. Since words have been demonstrated to be associated with the creative process, you have just discovered the mechanism by which your world is partially constructed. You have also just experienced manifestation in action.

The second major pathway of access for reconstructing the database of creative manifestation is that of observing your thoughts. Now, this is less frequently employed, and somewhat more tedious a task in that it requires another style of discipline. Most people are unfamiliar with how to observe

Your 60,000 Daily Thoughts

- The words you speak represent your thoughts.
- The two methods of modifying thought are awareness of the mechanism and observation of your thoughts.
- Breathing, meditation, prayer, contemplation, and affirmation directly impact the virtual.
- The two major pathways of access to the virtual are recognition and practice.

their own thoughts, or they are unwilling to engage in or maintain this type of practice. Remember that failure, in addition to being the discovery of how something doesn't work, is propagated by a lack of desire and commitment to a system that does work. Both of these approaches are fundamental systems for identifying the factors causing repeated symptoms to arise from the unseen realm. The goal in addressing these factors is to create a purposeful authenticity that allows you to be in the world, but not of it, and exist in an ever-present awareness.

Initiating a discipline to assist in achieving the conscious creation of your thoughts is simply a matter of intending to do that and choosing a way in which to accomplish it. There are as many ways as there are people. However, for the purpose of our present discussion, I'll share a few of the more common, popular, and historically effective.

■ Prescription for Change

Following your decision to initiate a practice designed to assist you in observing your thoughts, it is important to establish a regular time and place for performing it. While any consistent activity that you enjoy can serve the general purpose of stress-relief and relaxation, certain techniques provide for a permanent alteration of the processes that contribute to the need for relieving stress. In other words, it's good to have a way to release the accumulated effects of stress in your life. But, it's better to adopt a technique that allows for the created stresses to be minimized or eliminated in the first place.

Abraham Maslow, a prominent psychologist during the mid-twentieth century, introduced a model of developmental psychology that has become extremely well known not only in the field of psychology, but also in management and other human sciences. It describes five developmental stages, which are based on what Maslow calls human needs. Thus, his model is known as Maslow's Needs Hierarchy. In his later years, he expanded his model to include the higher levels of human experience.

Dr. C. George Boeree produced a biography of Maslow called *Personality Theories* from which I paraphrase the following details of Maslow's philosophy. Maslow explains that the human has five levels of needs, which build one upon the other. To develop a next higher level requires a reasonable level of completion, wholeness, integration, or stability at the previous level or levels. When this relative completion of a stage occurs, the desire or longing for the

202 ■ Beyond Medicine

next higher level automatically emerges over time. His initial list of needs included the following:

- **Physiological Needs:** These are the primary needs, which include the needs for food, water, air, and sleep. Without these, physical life itself is not possible.
- **Safety Needs:** Once the physiological needs are met, there are the needs for a safe lifestyle and safe environments. These might include safe housing, financial security, job security, as well as physical, mental, and emotional safety and freedom from threats.
- **Social Needs:** Beyond the safety needs arise the needs for belonging, such as having family, friends, and community. It involves the giving and receiving of love and nurturing.
- **Esteem Needs:** With social needs intact, the needs for self-respect, achievement, and recognition by others follow. Maslow later modified this somewhat, by explaining that between these esteem needs and the need for self-actualization, there is also the need for aesthetics and knowledge.
- **Self-Actualization:** The culmination of Maslow's original needs hierarchy is that of attaining one's full potential as a human being living in the world, involving the seeking and expression of justice, wisdom, benevolence, and creativity.

In his later years, Maslow added a sixth level to his needs hierarchy, that of "transcendence or transpersonal." This was in recognition of realities that are "trans," or beyond, all of the first five levels, including even the fifth stage of self-actualization. It is very important to note that there is a great difference between the terms self-actualization and self-realization. The former has to do with higher levels of fulfillment at the personality level but still in relation to worldliness. Self-realization has to do with that knowing of pure consciousness, which is beyond, transcendent, or transpersonal.

■ Meditation Means Awareness

Ultimately, the most productive form of practice is going to revolve around some form of meditation. Meditation means awareness. Whatever you do with awareness is meditation. Watching your breath is meditation; listening to the birds is meditation. As long as these activities are free from any other distraction to the mind, it is effective meditation.

All forms of meditation can be considered as a form of yoga. Yoga is the mastery and integration of the activities of mind. For that reason, it is frequently defined as union. Yoga is not merely physical fitness, stress management, medical treatment, or a technique for manifesting your desires; although authentic yoga is definitely beneficial to many aspects of life. Students of yoga meditation have different inclinations toward the practice stages of preparation, hatha yoga or stretches, relaxation, breathing, and meditation. Some may like to spend a long time on body work, while others prefer breathing exercises, and still others seek the stillness of meditation. Each of these stages work together, one leading into the next. There is no perfect, one-size-fits-all formula in meditation. It is best to spend the amount of time with each stage that is just right for you.

According to yoga psychology, presented by American-born Swami Jnaneshvara Bharati, there are three additional levels of development, experience, or being, which are beyond the five primary needs designated by Maslow. Eventually, even these three levels sequentially emerge as needs, as the longing for deeper and deeper truths intensifies. Just as with Maslow's five stages, each of these is sought one after the other. At first, one might seek the subtle, including any of the familiar objects, such as visualized images, sensation, breath, mantra, and attitudes, etc. Then one begins to realize that there is more. The focus changes to more formless insights, closer to the cause of creation. This focus might include the subtler components of those familiar objects sought after in the first level. The focus of attention shifts to the process and instruments by which observing or seeking is done. Then, even that is desired to be transcended, seeking nothing less than a direct experience or realization of absolute reality, truth, self, or union with God. Here, attention has shifted not only past the first level objects and their subtle elements, but also the sensory and mental processes by which they were being observed. Attention is now directed towards the observer itself, seeking to experience the subtlest aspect of individuation.

According to Swami Jnaneshvara, meditation is a systematic process that moves through stages. Meditation may begin with a gross object that has shape and form. Gradually, the meditation may deepen into the subtler aspects of that object. Systematically, attention then explores the mental and sensory instruments by which that gross object is observed, experienced, and understood. Then, the individual observer itself becomes the focus of exploration. Finally, the reality beyond the objects, the observing process, and the observer is experienced.

The various styles and forms of meditation practices are uniquely personal. In the beginning, it is best to avoid complicated techniques that might discourage you from continuing with the practice. In fact, an effective initial approach to establishing this discipline can be accomplished in as little as three minutes a day. For example, Swami Jnaneshvara describes the activities involved in a three-minute meditation. They are timed approximately like this: Take fifteen seconds to achieve a comfortable sitting position. Take the next forty-five seconds to survey the body. Allow your attention to gently move internally, through yourself, as you observe areas of discomfort or tension. Next, be aware of the breath at the diaphragm, just below the rib cage. Explore the breath as if you are really curious. For the next thirty seconds initiate diaphragmatic breathing, eliminating jerks and pauses, and making your breath steady, smooth, and comfortably slow. For the next thirty seconds initiate spinal breathing. Breathe as though exhaling down from the top of the head to the base of the spine. Inhale as though inhaling up from the base of the spine to the top of the head. Finally, bring attention to your breath at the bridge of the nostrils, feeling the touch of the air. For the next sixty seconds meditate by bringing awareness to your breath at the nostrils.

The purpose is to train your own ability to direct attention, which is the primary tool of meditation. After the three minutes, you may find you are relaxed and want to be still beyond the time of this practice. Regardless of the style or form of practice that you adopt, the basic approach to the entire process includes the following:

1. Relax the body.
2. Sit in a comfortable, straight, steady posture.
3. Make your breathing process serene.
4. Witness objects traveling through your mind.
5. Inspect the quality of your thoughts.
6. Promote thoughts that are helpful.
7. Do not allow yourself to be disturbed in any situation.
8. Let the skills you develop work together to deepen your awareness.

Once you have disciplined yourself to this basic practice, you can begin to explore new techniques, pursue additional skills, and extend the amount of time that you perform these techniques. As you become more adept at the basic procedures, you can begin to refine each element of the process according to your personal preferences.

Thoughts for Living

- What you focus on expands.
- Attention creates intention.
- Intention produces action.
- Action produces experience.
- Experience produces desire.

For instance, at the time of meditation you may choose to become aware of the external world, however broad that may be for you: universe, galaxy, Earth, country, city, home. Gradually you can bring your attention closer from the vast, external world, to the nearby world of your daily life, finally coming to the space your body is occupying.

Next, you could become aware of your ability to move, but that you are not moving; of grasping, but that you are letting go; of speaking, but of not now forming words. You can then become aware of the five senses of smell, taste, seeing, touching, and hearing. Close the doors called senses, and bring your attention inward.

Next, you can perform a more comprehensive survey of the body from head to toe and toe to head. Do this systematically; so that the path you follow each time is similar, though the experience may be different. However you experience the body is OK: parts, systems, and sensations. Again, do this as if you are really curious about exploring within as an interior researcher.

Next, be aware of the process of mind, allowing streams of thoughts to flow naturally, as you observe your breath. Bring attention to the area of your heart or to the center of your eyebrows. Continuing to allow thoughts to flow will assist in cultivating two skills: remaining focused in the space, while at the same time letting go of the thought patterns.

Next, allow your attention to go deep into the stillness and silence that surrounds you. Bring your attention to the chosen object of your meditation. As your meditation deepens, survey your internal space for the invisible source of all light, or listen into that space for the silent source of all sound.

Allow the inner peace or spiritual truth that emerges to come forward without judgment or resistance.

When you finish your meditation, bring that deep stillness and silence with you into the activities of your day.

■ Converting Cause

The underlying apparatus of these systems for identifying the factors causing repeated symptoms to arise from the unseen realm consists of the field
of energy and information I have referred to throughout this book. You
access both of these through your attention with the intention of transforming their potential into tangible life experiences. To convert potential into
probability, you must access the fertile soil between established thought
patterns. To do this, you must plant new seeds of expectation fertilized by
your intention for new experiences. You must then nurture these new seeds
by consistently watering them with sustained attention to the words that
you speak. In so doing, you will begin to recreate your reality as an expression of your innate, genetic purpose and passion.

Both of these techniques will work and are extremely effective for
reconfiguring the software of the unseen into a more productive format. In
addition, there are literally hundreds of enhancement tools for refining and
expediting this process. In addition to the practices of meditation, contemplation, and prayer, there is one called mantra. A mantra is a word or sound
that is repeated over and over for a specific period of time. This practice
can be used as means of relieving the autonomic nervous system, while
calming and focusing the mind. Mantra practice like this will prepare the
mind for deeper meditation. All of these practices can assist in establishing
clarity, will, focus, and surrender. But again, selecting something that is
compatible and effective will be key in terms of your long-term commitment, compliance, and results.

■ Designing with Words

When choosing to initiate the practice of working with words as a means
for renovating your reality, you might elect to use a simple reminder technique, such as a rubber band around your wrist. Every time you verbalize
expressions that contribute to keeping you where you are, you immediately
become aware of the significance and snap the rubber band on your wrist
to encourage yourself to be more aware. You then can begin substituting
alternative verbal expressions. Usually, within thirty days of beginning this
practice, you will notice a marked improvement in the language you speak,
or you will have one very red wrist.

As a side benefit to employing this technique, you will quickly see that the nature of your relationships and daily interactions begin to improve. As you become more conscious of the words you select to communicate, you will also begin to become less reactive and more responsive. Subsequently, you will begin to realize that the situations and circumstances with which you are confronted no longer dictate your behavior. In effect, they will begin to present you with opportunities to incorporate them into your master plan for achieving and accomplishing your goal of peaceful and productive existence.

Affirmations are also a productive tool to use in conjunction with the rubber band method of modifying spoken words. Prayer can be a form of affirmation, if used correctly. Remember, you ask and receive not, because you ask amiss. So the way you construct your prayers, affirmations, and positive statements will have a tremendous effect on the results you obtain.

■ Constructing Requests

There are two major obstacles to properly constructing requests of the unseen. The first is asking the wrong way. An example would be requests beginning with I want or I need. All this does is perpetuate lack in that you have prefaced your request with the want or need as the object of your request. In other words, using language such as I want or I need simply suggests that you don't have and are actually asking for more want or need.

The second obstacle is a properly constructed request with which you fail to maintain an attitude of gratitude or belief that you will actually receive what you have requested. When you submit to the universe a gimme attitude, the universe will respond with a hundred fold gimme and take even more from you. When you extend gratefulness for having received that which you are requesting, you will receive more than you asked for in your initial appeal. Remember, to remain viable, your request must come from a place of believing that you already have what you've asked for, as suggested by the verse from Hebrews 11:1 (NKJV): "Faith is the substance of things asked for and the evidence of things not yet seen."

All of the tools beyond these two major pathways of access will simply serve to compliment, refine, and enhance your efforts. You can vary them, combine them, quit them, modify them, or incorporate them into a focused and intense commitment to experience whatever you choose. I'm not going to detail the specific mechanisms by which each of these contributes to your ultimate goal. I will merely present a short list of the more common options for observing and modifying Repetitive Thought Disorders.

■ Repetitive Thought Repair

The most effective and productive methods for working directly with your thought pool entail tools such as meditation, contemplation, and prayer. All of these are similar in that they direct your attention to the existing competition in the thought realm. This creates an awareness of what you're currently working with in this unseen realm. In concentrating your attention on this influential realm, you can begin to observe the nature of its dynamics, while engaging an opportunity for modifying its content.

One of the most efficient and useful techniques for accomplishing this involves only about twenty minutes of your time. This can be done in the morning, evening, or both. The technique entails taking some quiet, undisturbed time to sit quietly, while focusing on your breathing pattern of inhalation and exhalation. Directing your awareness exclusively to your breath provides you with the opportunity to simply observe the thoughts that arise, while allowing them to freely pass through your consciousness. The net effect is a slowing down of the thought process. This creates fewer distractive thoughts with more space in between them. This provides you an opportunity to introduce deliberate thoughts consistent with what you have chosen to experience.

■ Supplementary Techniques

Some ancillary techniques that can be used in conjunction with this technique include the verbalism of sounds that I referred to earlier, called mantras. The inclusion of this technique can help further focus and direct your attention to the intention at hand. On the website, www.swamij.com "Yoga Meditation of the Himalayan Tradition," two specific forms of this technique are described. They are called Japa and Ajapa-Japa. Japa means repeating or remembering the mantra. Ajapa-Japa means constant awareness. The letter A in front of the word Japa means without. Thus, Ajapa-Japa is the practice of Japa without the mental effort normally needed to repeat the mantra. In other words, it has become automatic, turning into a constant awareness. The practice of constant remembrance evolves in stages.

At first, you intentionally repeat the syllables of the mantra as if you are talking to yourself in your mind. You allow the inner sound to come at whatever speed feels comfortable to your mind. With practice, the mantra is repeated automatically, like a song that you have heard many times, which just comes on its own. Gradually, you merely remember the mantra with attention drawn to it. It is more like noticing what is already happening, rather than causing it to happen. It is somewhat like the attention stance of listening rather than speaking, though you might not literally hear the sound.

In time, the feeling of the mantra is there, even when the sound or remembering of the syllables is not there. For example, sometimes people will say, "Om, shanti, shanti, shanti," where the word shanti means peace or tranquility. During the remembering of the word, there may be two things— the word and the feeling of peace or tranquility. When the syllables fade away, the feeling may still be there as a remembrance of the feeling of the mantra. As the practice evolves, there comes a pervasive awareness of the mantra, subtler than both the syllables and any surface level meaning or definition. This constant awareness is the meaning of Ajapa-Japa of the mantra.

There are many mantras, words, or compact prayers that can be used for Japa and Ajapa-Japa. Virtually all of the meditation traditions, spiritual lineages, and religions have mantra in one form or another. Some words have specific meaning, while others are associated only with a feeling. They are not literal translations with specific definitions. Some have religious significance, while others are completely non-sectarian. Some have very subtle effects on energy, while others are more like positive affirmations given to train the conscious mind.

As you progress and further utilize this technique, your selection of sounds will become more specific. You will realize that the vibration associated with the sound produces a calm clarity because of its high frequency and creative characteristics. The laws that govern this phenomenon dictate that everything vibrates and everything moves. In general, the faster the vibration, the closer you come to resonating with the consciousness that creates and sustains all of existence. Conversely, slower vibrations keep you closer to the slow moving world of the physical and the problems associated with material existence. By using a mantra you become more sensitive and receptive to frequencies carrying the solutions of interpretation, insight, and creativity.

You alone can choose to eliminate whatever it is that prevents or restricts you from increasing your vibratory output by employing any of the techniques presented in this chapter for moving into a more profound relationship with your source energy. In fact, you can solicit the help you are seeking by simply asking, trusting, and knowing that the best possible response has been provided, even before you ask.

■ Recapitulation

Another powerful technique for altering your experience at the level where thoughts originate is called recapitulation. This is a form of self-therapy in which you relive the day that has just passed on the inner screen of your conscious awareness. See your day from the moment of awakening to the moment you sit down with yourself to review the events. This is a very effective way of objectively assessing your strengths, weaknesses, ideals, goals, and behaviors. There is no need to judge, analyze, or evaluate. Simply observe, file it away for future reference, if need be, and forget it. This simple process alone will gradually and subtly affect the dynamics of your day-to-day interactions.

If you're feeling adventurous or just bored, you can kick it up a notch and do the same thing with your dreams, attempting to recall them in detail before you engage the day. Oftentimes, keeping a journal near your bed will prove to be helpful in recalling some of the more memorable events, and provide insight and guidance for the day ahead.

In the final analysis, to effectively engage a productive interaction of all of the realms, you must adopt conscious and consistent tools for working with each of them and monitoring the outcomes. There is no success or failure when it comes to a self-help program of this nature, only results. Remember, everything works. So pick a name, choose a formula, initiate a discipline, and the journey begins.

Seek out tools that interest you, apply them, experiment, explore and remember that your ever-present awareness will dictate your life experience, so seek first to be ever-present.

"Since you become what you embody, you are fostering a self-fulfilling prophecy!"

—LAURA DAY, THE CIRCLE

Appendix

"The great aim of education is not knowledge but action."

—HERBERT SPENCER, ENGLISH PHILOSOPHER (1820–1903)

Some Things to Remember

Caveats to guide your decisions:
- Anything can cause anything.
- For every action, there is a reaction.
- Everything works.
- There are no panaceas.
- When all you have is a hammer, everything looks like a nail.
- When you hear hoof beats, look for horses.
- Everything is what it isn't.

Some things to reflect on:
- Now is the time to begin because there is no time but now.
- Anything can cause anything, so how do you know what's causing what?

- You get what you give, so give what you want to receive.
- Expectation is 90 percent of manifestation.
- Words bring your expectations into your experience.
- As you think, so will be your experience of life.
- The instructions you follow determine the reality you create.
- The only thing you can do for anyone else is work on yourself.
- Your outcome is only as good as the system you employ.
- What you experience is not nearly as important as how you experience it.
- The best predictor of future behavior is past behavior.
- When you choose the behavior, you choose the consequences.
- When you change the way you look at things, the things you look at change.

Other key concepts to ponder:
- The main thing that's wrong is that you think something's wrong.
- Nothing happens until something moves.
- Successful results depend on desire, commitment, and a system that works.
- You are ultimately responsible for everything you experience.
- What you focus on expands.
- Attention creates intention.
- Intention produces action.
- Action produces experience.
- Experience produces desire.

Integrating the Realms

The Physical Realm

Exercise:
- Motion is life.
- Exercise is essential.
- Choose something you like and can commit to.
- Cross-train regularly.
- Look for exercise that combines flexibility, strength, balance, and endurance.
- Take time to relax and recover.

Nutrition:

- Find a diet that works for you.
- Adopt a diet that fits your lifestyle.
- Pay attention to cravings and related symptoms.
- Diversify regularly.

The Biochemical Realm:

- Everyone must take five specific supplements daily: a broad spectrum multiple vitamin, a comprehensive mineral complex, an antioxidant, a probiotic and a digestive enzyme.
- Additional supplements are required on an individual basis.
- Nutritional testing is essential to developing a comprehensive program.
- Our biochemistry is a bi-directional link between the physical and the virtual.

The Virtual Realm:

- You have 60,000 thoughts per day.
- The majority of thoughts are the same day after day.
- All thoughts arise in the present moment.
- Many thoughts are about past guilt and future anxiety.
- The space between thoughts is the soil for new thoughts.
- The nature of your thoughts will determine your life experience.
- The words you speak coagulate the influence of your thoughts.
- Repetitive Thought Disorders produce Vicious Cycle Disorders.
- Vicious Cycle Disorders are repeated patterns of behavior.
- Breathing, meditation, prayer, contemplation, and affirmation directly impact the virtual.
- The two major pathways of access to the virtual are recognition and practice.
- The two methods of modifying thought are awareness of the mechanism and observation of our thoughts.

Other Notions to Entertain:

- Life is tri-dimensional.
- Existence is multidimensional.
- An imbalance in one realm creates imbalance in the others.
- Diseases are symptoms of an undiagnosed imbalance.
- You may not be sick, but you may be unwell.
- The essence of physical longevity is nutrients in and waste products out.
- Three major influences shaping reality are genetics, environment, and stress.
- Identifying cause is the cure for symptoms.

A Final Word

The information upon which these tools for wellness are based is synthesized from my own experience over thirty years as a primary caregiver. This information is by no means all-inclusive, nor does it suggest that this is the only way to achieve your objectives. It is, however, representative of the core concepts upon which the general dynamics of human interaction occur.

Whole person therapy is the future of the healing arts. Our bodies are miraculous gifts and marvelously constructed vehicles that allow us the opportunity to express our innate divinity and the unlimited potential of all that the virtual realm represents. The choice of how to experience this inexplicable mystery remains yours. In choosing to be ever-present, your encounter will most certainly be "beyond medicine."

About the Author

With credentials in both the conventional and complementary care arenas, Dr. Richard DiCenso provides unique insight into the mysteries of the healing arts. Trained as an acupuncturist and a chiropractic physician, Dr. DiCenso maintains an active practice as the Clinical Director of Advanced Therapeutics in Virginia Beach, VA. Based upon his experience, training and approach to healthcare issues, he is considered to be an expert in "Whole Person Therapy." He lectures regularly to enthusiastic audiences on subjects as diverse as menopause, weight loss, proactive wellness, medical politics, lifestyle changes, forensics and nutritional biochemistry.

Dr. DiCenso has thirty years of experience managing the chronic symptoms of Vicious Cycle Disorders (VCD). He has been called upon to treat numerous professional athletes, celebrities, and healthcare professionals. Dr. DiCenso has also presented and developed wellness programs for the U.S. Government, Omega Institute, Kripalu Institute, The Option Institute, and Canyon Ranch.

Having served as Clinical Director and Program Administrator in several healthcare facilities across the country, Dr. DiCenso's primary focus is the elimination of symptom care. Using his extensive background in human biochemistry and orthomolecular nutrition, he has become one of the leading authorities in the field of biological fluid analysis. He has helped thousands of individuals around the world with undiagnosable symptoms to dramatically improve their health without drugs or surgery.

He is skilled as a forensic chiropractor and disability examiner, and is also an expert in the revolutionary science of manipulation under anesthesia. Dr. DiCenso maintains privileges at a number of hospitals throughout the country. Dr. DiCenso draws upon his extensive background in human biochemistry and nutrition to design wellness programs using the twenty-first century technology of Quantum Fluid Analysis and M.A.P. testing in his Virginia Beach Center. Dr. DiCenso also appears regularly in newspapers, on radio, on television, and in public forums supporting self-health awareness and the evolution of wellness.

Dr. DiCenso is available for speaking engagements and personal consults. For more information about Matrix Transformation, or to inquire about mail-order M.A.P. testing, please contact Dr. DiCenso's office at 1-800-959-2640, or visit his website at www.matrixtransformation.com.